8 Ways to Prevent Pancreatic Cancer

Other books by this author

- Microscopic Colitis (Available in English and Spanish)
- Understanding Microscopic Colitis
- Vitamin D and Autoimmune Disease

8 Ways to Prevent Pancreatic Cancer

Wayne Persky

Persky Farms

United States

First published and distributed in the United States of America by:
Persky Farms, 19242 Darrs Creek Rd, Bartlett, TX 76511-4022
Tel.: (1)254-527-3682, (1)254-718-1125
Email: wayne@perskyfarms.com

Disclaimer and Legal Notice: The information contained in this book is intended solely for general educational purposes, and is not intended, nor implied, to be a substitute for professional medical advice relative to any specific medical condition or question. The advice of a physician or other health care provider should always be sought for any questions regarding any medical condition. Specific diagnoses and therapies can only be provided by the reader's physician. The author and the publisher specifically disclaim any and all liability arising directly or indirectly from the use or application of any information contained in this book.

Please note that some of the information in this book is based on personal experience and anecdotal evidence. Although the author and publisher have made every reasonable attempt to achieve complete accuracy of the content, they assume no responsibility for errors or omissions. If you should choose to use any of this information, use it according to your best judgment, and at your own risk. Because your particular situation will not exactly match the examples upon which this information is based, you should adjust your use of the information and recommendations to fit your own personal situation.

This book does not recommend or endorse any specific tests, products, procedures, opinions, or other information that may be mentioned anywhere in the book. This information is provided for educational purposes, and reliance on any tests, products, procedures, or opinions mentioned in the book is solely at the reader's own risk. Any trademarks, service marks, product names, or named features are assumed to be the property of their respective owners, and are used only for reference. There is no implied endorsement when these terms are used in this book.

ISBN 978-0-9859772-4-5

This book is dedicated to everyone concerned about pancreatic cancer, and especially to everyone who has lost a loved one to the disease.

Table of Contents

Introduction

Pancreatic cancer is one of the deadliest forms of cancer known. According to most medical authorities, even if it happens to be diagnosed early, it still often has a poor prognosis because it tends to spread so rapidly. And seldom is it diagnosed early enough to be effectively treated. A diagnosis carries the seriousness of a death sentence in most cases because 80 % of pancreatic cancer patients survive less than a year, and only about 10 % survive past the second year. Only 6 % survive longer than 5 years.

Obviously this is a disease that everyone should be doing everything they possibly can to prevent becoming a victim. New evidence indicates that pancreatic cancer develops over a number of years. This suggests that like other types of cancer, pancreatic cancer may develop as a result of unresolved chronic health issues. Correcting those issues before cancer has time to develop may provide the best way to minimize the risk of developing the disease.

Fortunately there are a number of things that almost anyone can do that can make a significant difference in reducing the risk of developing pancreatic cancer. This book describes some of the ways that should be effective for helping to avoid becoming a victim of the disease.

You may be wondering, "Why don't our doctors tell us about this?" Probably because they either are not aware of this information, or because of either time limitations or liability concerns. Appointment scheduling is so tight these days that doctors can scarcely afford to waste any time if they are going to provide a reasonable standard of care for their patients. Hospital and clinic administrators are continually pushing physicians to see more patients each day. And legal departments especially discourage any behavior that does not follow "accepted medical policies". For a clinician to make recommendations to a patient that might not be considered to be part of "accepted medical policies" is sort of like volunteering information in court, or volunteering information when a traffic cop stops someone for speeding — there's little to be gained, and it can cause the case to be lost in court.

Currently, physicians have no approved methods for early screening for pancreatic cancer before clinical symptoms begin, and by the time clinical symptoms begin, the disease has typically already reached a stage at which it cannot be effectively treated. Published research articles such as those cited in this book are certainly available, so physicians could find the information if they choose to do so. But again, these days most physicians are so short of free time that they typically don't have adequate time available to do such research unless they have a specific and immediate need. It's time-consuming enough just complying with all the reporting requirements of the current health care program and the insurance companies, plus trying to keep up with all the new drugs that become available every year.

Although preventing future health problems has not been an emphasized part of most physicians' job description, there are signs that changes in this policy are being explored. And better understanding of genetic risks and diet essentials will eventually prepare physicians to be much more helpful for future health planning. But even if this trend becomes well established, it may be many years before enough progress is made that patients will be able to safely rely on their physicians to look out for all aspects of their long-term health. No one is perfect, and the human body is an extremely complex machine that no one truly understands.

In the meantime, patients must be willing to assume the responsibility for their own health, and they must stay informed and be willing to adopt lifestyle changes that offer the promise of improved long-term health. Taking steps to minimize the risk of developing deadly diseases such as pancreatic cancer should obviously be a part of that plan.

This book is relatively brief and it's focused on risk factors for pancreatic cancer that have been verified by published medical research. It can be read and understood in a relatively short amount of time. And the information in the book is organized so that it can be used as a quick reference when needed in the future. Cited references are listed in a bibliography at the end of the book so that more detailed information is readily available should anyone reading this book desire more information about specific topics.

Some of the evidence presented in this book is based on published medical research, some of it is based on interpretations and extrapolation of those research data, some of it is based on experience-based observations, aka epidemiological evidence, and some of the information is based on case studies. But the sources of that information are properly referenced, so that as you are reading you can judge for yourself whether these might be valid concerns for you. And you can decide which of these risks may be important enough that you definitely need to take action in order to minimize them, just to be on the safe side.

This book will help you to:
- Identify conditions that may put you at risk for pancreatic cancer
- Understand why these risks exist
- Rate the relative seriousness of the various risks
- Learn what to do to reduce those risks

Chapter 1

Mortality Rates are Extremely High for Pancreatic Cancer

Prevention is really the only practical approach because diagnosis and treatment continue to have very poor success rates.

Pancreatic cancer (PC) is typically diagnosed too late to be successfully treated. In most cases the tumor has already spread to other organs before any symptoms are noticed. Nor does it respond well to treatments using drugs or radiation. And even in many cases when it is thought to have been successfully surgically removed, as Gudjonsson (1987) pointed out, the cancer often reappears.[1] So it's no wonder that the prognosis is usually poor whenever PC is diagnosed.

Obviously that implies that the most effective way to prevent becoming another mortality statistic of the disease is to minimize the risk of developing it in the first place. Reducing the risk may actually be much easier than is commonly recognized, especially when compared with how overwhelmed the medical approach seems to be when dealing with pancreatic cancer.

According to Johns Hopkins University, pancreatic cancer is ranked as the fourth leading cancer in terms of deaths due to cancer (The Sol Goldman Pancreatic Cancer Research Center, 2015).[2] By 2020 it is predicted to be the second leading cause of deaths due to cancer (Imaging Technology News, 2012, November 9).[3] To add insult to injury, the U. S. government spends very little money on research devoted to pancreatic cancer, so it's not likely that the effectiveness of treatments for pancreatic cancer will significantly improve in the foreseeable future.

Note that pancreatic cancer is primarily a disease of adults.

As Dall'igna et al. (2010) concluded, medical statistics show that pediatric pancreatic cancer is extremely rare.[4] By the time you finish this book, you will understand why pediatric cancer is so rare. Although this observation is strictly speculation, the fact that pediatric cases are so rare provides support for the theory that pancreatic cancer is basically a disease caused by long-term dietary habits, rather than genetic issues. That said, genetic links may certainly exist, but they may play a subordinate role to dietary influences.

And that theory is the primary reason for writing this book.

Based on available research data, diet currently appears to be the most powerful weapon available for preventing pancreatic cancer. Basically, anyone can significantly increase their odds of preventing pancreatic cancer in most cases by simply correcting certain nutritional deficiencies and related diet risks that are common in most diets today that are based on the so-called Western diet. Doing so will not only greatly reduce the chances of developing pancreatic cancer, but correcting these deficiencies can provide many other health benefits that can help to prevent the development of other health problems in the future, thereby improving long-term health and quality of life.

The goal of this book is to acquaint the reader with the known risks associated with the development of pancreatic cancer so that those risks can be minimized, thereby preventing the disease from ever developing. These are risks that have been discovered by medical researchers and described in peer-reviewed, published medical research articles.

This will be a very short chapter. It's purpose is to list the most important health factors that have been identified by medical researchers to be associated with an increased risk of developing pancreatic cancer. The chapters that follow will discuss these respective associations and risks in detail.

Some of the health risks associated with pancreatic cancer include:

1. Magnesium deficiency
2. Diabetes
3. Vitamin D deficiency
4. Certain oral bacteria, specifically Porphyromonas gingivalis and Aggregatibacter actinomycetemcomitans
5. Poultry (yes, believe it or not, the same poultry that have been promoted for decades as a healthier protein choice than beef and pork)
6. Soy
7. Sugar, particularly fructose — this includes not only corn syrup and high-fructose corn syrup, but also fruit and fruit juices
8. Fat in the diet, particularly animal fat

There are other factors that have some effect, but many of them fall under the categories listed above. For example, obesity is thought to be associated with an increased risk of developing pancreatic cancer, but this may be due to the fact that obesity increases the risk of insulin resistance and the development of type 2 diabetes. And as we shall see in chapter 3, diabetes links back to magnesium deficiency.

And surely there are other risks that have not yet been discovered by medical researchers, that may come to light in the future. But based on current knowledge, the issues discussed in this book have been shown by medical research to be significantly associated with the risk of developing pancreatic cancer. And fortunately there are simple diet and lifestyle choices that can be made to take advantage of this information and thereby reduce the risk of developing PC.

Summary

Pancreatic cancer is currently ranked as the fourth leading cause of cancer deaths. By the year 2020 it is predicted to be the second leading cause of cancer deaths. Certain diet and health issues have been shown to significantly increase the risk of developing PC. The key to avoiding becoming another pancreatic cancer victim may lie in correcting those diet and health issues before PC has a chance to become established.

Chapter 2

Hypomagnesemia Is a Major Risk Factor for Pancreatic Cancer

It has been reported that most people are magnesium deficient, and this is one risk that is not only easy to correct, but resolving it often provides many other health benefits.

Hypomagnesemia is the medical term used to describe magnesium deficiency. In 2015, a very interesting study based on data collected between the years of 2000–2008, and focused on the use of magnesium supplements, was published by Dibaba, Xun, Yokota, White, and He.[5] The research project involved 66,806 men and women aged 50–76 years at the beginning of the study. The subjects in the study were ranked according to the percentage of magnesium supplement taken relative to the recommended daily allowance (RDA).

According to the official guidelines published by the U. S. government-affiliated National Institutes of Health, the RDA for men in this age range is 420 mg and the RDA for women in this age range is 320 mg (Magnesium Fact Sheet for Health Professionals, 2016, February 11).[6]

Bear in mind that the RDA amounts are intended to include the total amount of magnesium available from all sources, and for many people that amount might be limited to the magnesium content of food in their diet, while for others it might include both food and magnesium supplements. But this particular study ignored the magnesium content of food in the subjects' diet. It focused only on magnesium supplements.

With that in mind, the results published by Dibaba, Xun, Yokota, White, and He (2015) showed that compared with those who took the full RDA, those who took from 75–99 % of the RDA had a 42 % increased risk of developing pancreatic cancer. Those who took less than 75 % of the RDA showed a 76 % increased risk of developing pancreatic cancer. These results represent a very strong correlation.

Based on that study, taking a full RDA of magnesium supplement cuts the risk of pancreatic cancer in half.

According to the study results, every 100 mg per day decrease in magnesium supplement intake (below the RDA) was associated with a 24 % increase in the incidence of pancreatic cancer. Doing the math, that implies that women who took no magnesium supplement had approximately a 77 % increased risk, and men who took no magnesium supplement had slightly more than a 100 % increased risk. Together, on the average, that translates into roughly twice the risk of those who took a full RDA of magnesium supplement. Remember that this isn't just a projected rate — it's the actual increased rate at which pancreatic cancer developed among the group of people in this study.

So these research data suggest that anyone not currently taking a magnesium supplement can cut their risk of developing pancreatic cancer approximately in half simply by taking a magnesium supplement that meets the RDA guidelines. And according to the report, this relationship held true regardless of age, gender, body mass index, or non-steroidal anti-inflammatory drug (NSAID) use. From this observation one could possibly infer that the daily use of an NSAID (aspirin), probably provides no protection against pancreatic cancer, despite the claims made that regular aspirin use can help to prevent colon cancer.

Looking at the macroscopic implications of the findings of this research, it's painfully clear that a heck of a lot of people are magnesium-deficient these days. Otherwise, taking a full RDA of magnesium supplement should not have had such a profound effect on pancreatic cancer risk. Another way of looking at these data results might be to infer that perhaps the RDA listed for magnesium is only half of the amount actually needed for good health. At least that appears to be the case if avoiding diseases such as pancreatic cancer is considered to be a part of good health.

Remember, the study did not even consider the magnesium contained in the food in the diet of the subjects studied. It only looked at the amount of magnesium supplements they used.

According to the Magnesium Fact Sheet for Health Professionals published by the National Institutes of Health (cited on the first page of this chapter as reference number 6), here are the vital statistics on magnesium for normal human health. Notice the last sentence in the quote (emphasized here with bold print), which verifies that the blood tests typically used by doctors to measure magnesium levels are basically worthless unless the body is almost completely out of magnesium, which is a dangerous condition.

> *An adult body contains approximately 25 g magnesium, with 50% to 60% present in the bones and most of the rest in soft tissues. Less than 1% of total magnesium is in blood serum, and these levels are kept under tight control. Normal serum magnesium concentrations range be-*

tween 0.75 and 0.95 millimoles (mmol)/L. Hypomagnesemia is defined as a serum magnesium level less than 0.75 mmol/L. Magnesium homeostasis is largely controlled by the kidney, which typically excretes about 120 mg magnesium into the urine each day. Urinary excretion is reduced when magnesium status is low.

Assessing magnesium status is difficult because most magnesium is inside cells or in bone. ***The most commonly used and readily available method for assessing magnesium status is measurement of serum magnesium concentration, even though serum levels have little correlation with total body magnesium levels or concentrations in specific tissues.***

So with less than 1 % of the body's magnesium available in blood serum, it shouldn't be surprising that the blood tests typically used by doctors are almost worthless for assessing magnesium levels in the body. According to Mauskop and Varughese, (2012), approximately 67 % of the body's supply of magnesium is located in bone tissue, but that magnesium is pretty much unavailable for routine testing purposes.[7] And approximately 31 % is stored in cells.

A blood test is available for measuring the amount of magnesium available in red blood cells (known as the RBC magnesium test), but despite the fact that this test is much more accurate than the standard serum test, it's rarely ordered because it's a more complex test than the serum test. The most accurate magnesium blood test is a test known as the ionized magnesium test. But unfortunately this test is not available to most people because it is only available at a few select locations.

The most accurate magnesium test of all is known as an EXA test. EXA stands for Energy Dispersive X-Ray Analysis. This test is based on tissue samples scraped from the mouth. But similar to the ionized magnesium test, finding a physician or a lab set up to do the EXA test can be difficult.

All magnesium supplements are not created equal.

Magnesium comes in many different forms (compounds) and some forms are much more easily absorbed than others. Unabsorbed magnesium remains in the intestines along with other waste material, and if the amount of magnesium supplement taken is large enough, and absorption is poor, the unabsorbed magnesium can act as a laxative.

For example, magnesium oxide is poorly absorbed. Typically, only about 2–4 % of magnesium oxide is absorbed into the bloodstream. It's the cheapest form of magnesium available, and not surprisingly, it has the poorest absorption characteristics of all the available options. When water is added to magnesium oxide, the result is magnesium hydroxide, otherwise known as milk of magnesia, a common laxative. So obviously one wouldn't want to take very much magnesium oxide unless the goal is to resolve a constipation problem. The point is, magnesium oxide is an extremely poor choice when attempting to resolve a magnesium deficiency. Much better forms, with better absorption characteristics are available.

One of the most easily absorbed forms of magnesium that's commonly available is chelated magnesium (aka magnesium glycinate).

Magnesium glycinate is also one of the more expensive forms of magnesium (not surprisingly). And this form of magnesium is one of the least-likely forms to cause diarrhea when larger doses are used. Magnesium glycinate is a chelation of magnesium and glycine, an amino acid. Because amino acids are readily absorbed in the small intestine, magnesium glycine is readily absorbed.

But beware of products sold as "Buffered" Chelated Magnesium because in many cases the buffering agent appears to be simply cheap magnesium oxide. And in such products magnesium oxide may be used to replace up to 50 % of the chelated magnesium.

Rather than being an enhancement, an addition of this sort behaves more like an adulteration of the product. The buyer mistakenly believes that the manufacturer is looking out for her or his welfare by considerately adding a "buffering" agent to enhance absorption efficiency or safety, when in fact all that the manufacturer is doing is ripping off the customer by selling cheap magnesium oxide at chelated magnesium prices. And of course the magnesium oxide can undo the benefits of chelated magnesium by significantly reducing the amount of magnesium that will be likely to be absorbed, and this can increase the chances that larger doses might promote diarrhea in some cases. Up to 50 % of the elemental magnesium in magnesium glycinate can be absorbed. However, if half the magnesium glycinate is replaced by magnesium oxide, then the amount of magnesium likely to be absorbed will be approximately cut in half.

Magnesium citrate often works satisfactorily. As long as the amount taken does not significantly exceed the RDA, most types of magnesium (other than magnesium oxide) should not cause diarrhea except in unusual cases, or when large doses are taken.

Topically-applied magnesium oil or lotion is another option.

In cases where oral magnesium supplements are not well-tolerated, topical applications (on the skin) can be used instead. When magnesium oils or lotions are applied to the skin, the magnesium is readily absorbed and stored in the cells in muscle tissue and other organs where it will be available when needed by the body. Some people leave magnesium oil or lotion in place after it soaks in, while others prefer to apply it 20 or 30 minutes before taking a bath or shower. For spray products, it's usually best to spray it into the palm of one's hand and then rub it on the skin, because any spray that misses the mark and lands on the floor can create slick spots that can cause someone to slip and fall.

Foot soaks in Epsom salts are also effective.

And adding Epsom salts to bath water is another way to increase one's daily intake of magnesium. Some people prefer to use a combination of oral supplementation and topical applications in order to get an adequate dose without upsetting their digestive system. This can be especially helpful in cases where the digestive system is already sensitive due to other issues.

One thing to watch out for that causes many people to unintentionally take half as much magnesium as they intend to take is a very misleading labeling practice that is often used for oral magnesium supplements. Many manufacturers show the amount of magnesium on the front label as the "serving size" dose rather than the dose per tablet. In other words, if for example the label shows 400 mg on the front label, one would normally assume that this means that each tablet contains 400 mg of magnesium. But that may not be the case.

Unfortunately, in many cases a careful review of the back label will reveal that the product actually contains 400 mg "per serving", and somewhere on the back label the "serving size" will be specified as 2 tablets. In other words, each tablet contains only half the amount displayed on the front label, which would be 200 mg in this example. This is a very misleading practice, but it isn't true for all magnesium supplement products — some actually contain the amount specified on the front label in each tablet. So be sure to read both labels carefully when selecting a product and determining the proper dose.

Don't allow yourself to be tricked into taking half enough magnesium.

Remember that according to the research study described earlier in this chapter, accidentally taking only half the RDA can increase the risk of developing pancreatic cancer by approximately 50 %. Labels should always be carefully read, not simply scanned. This is very important.

But improved protection against pancreatic cancer may not be the biggest advantage of supplementing with magnesium. Sadly, many cases of hypertension are actually due to undiagnosed magnesium deficiency. Therefore, if you are taking any blood pressure medications, please be aware that you may need to discuss reducing your medication dosage with your doctor, or possibly discontinue taking it altogether as you slowly resolve your magnesium deficiency after using magnesium supplements for a while.

It may take months or even years of supplementation before magnesium reserves can be rebuilt to the point where blood pressure is significantly reduced, but magnesium is so effective at reducing blood pressure that many authorities caution against using too much magnesium and reducing one's blood pressure too much. That's not likely to happen unless very large doses are taken (2 or 3 times the RDA or more) or kidney function is compromised. Excess magnesium is removed from circulation by the kidneys and eliminated from the body in urine. Reduced kidney function can lead to a dangerous buildup of magnesium in circulation, and taking excessively large doses of magnesium can impose an increased workload on the kidneys.

Therefore if you happen to have kidney disease or other issues that cause compromised kidney function, be sure to check with your doctor before beginning a magnesium supplementation program. Normally though, unless magnesium supplementation rates significantly exceed the RDA, supplementing with magnesium will simply bring one's systolic blood pressure down to where it actually should be in the absence of a magnesium deficiency.

Most people believe that they eat a healthy (nutritious) diet.

They read labels on processed foods and they try to eat a balanced diet. The "health police" climb down from their ivory towers occasionally to assure everyone that following their recommendations will ensure good health. But out in the real world, it's impossible to ignore the fact that more and more people are developing allergies and food sensitivities and autoimmune diseases and cancer and various other health issues. So why isn't all the "expert" health advice working?

Is it possible that our foods might not be as nutritious as they are thought to be?

And could it be that some of the official RDA guidelines for vitamins and minerals are simply wrong, and they significantly understate optimal values for good health for many people? One of the serious problems with the RDA guidelines is that they assume that all people absorb nutrients at some arbitrary "normal" rate. RDA guidelines consider age, gender, pregnancy, and a few other categories. But in the real world, even within those categories, everyone does not absorb nutrients at that so-called "normal" rate. Nutrient absorption can vary widely, depending upon genetics, gut bacteria profiles, digestive health issues, disease, general health, physical activity levels, and other conditions that can compromise absorption.

13

Numerous published research reports show that certain RDA listings are not consistent with current research. For example, compelling epidemiological evidence indicates that the RDA listings for vitamin D are only adequate for preventing the development of the disease known as rickets. Far higher blood levels of vitamin D are necessary for preventing the development of most other diseases (Persky, 2013, pp. 87–88).[8] This will be explored in more detail in chapter 4.

And what about items in our diet that deplete magnesium?

Some of the foods we eat or drink are known to deplete certain nutrients, but it appears that issues such as these are totally ignored by the RDA guidelines. The guidelines assume that everyone eats and drinks basically the same foods. But does a one-size-fits-all approach actually work?

Coffee depletes magnesium.

And the more coffee one consumes, the more magnesium will likely be lost. This suggests that if one drinks more coffee than most people in the general population, then more magnesium intake than normal may be needed. It's easy to assume that a single extra cup of coffee shouldn't make a significant difference. And that's true, it probably won't. But an extra cup of coffee every day will definitely make a significant difference, and that difference could result in a long-term magnesium deficiency in some cases. Alcohol is also known to deplete magnesium (Flink, 1986).[9]

Many medications deplete magnesium.

The list includes various types of medications including corticosteroids, certain antibiotics, antacids, contraceptives, cardiovascular medications. diuretics, proton pump inhibitors, and possibly others. These medications don't necessarily totally prevent the absorption of magnesium, and their effects can vary among individuals, but in most cases they reduce the amount of magnesium absorbed enough to cause a significant reduction in magnesium levels. They can negatively affect both short term blood levels of magnesium and magnesium reserves that are stored in cells for future use.

As an example of how serious the problem of drugs interfering with the absorption of magnesium can be, consider the first paragraph of a warning issued by the FDA regarding the use of proton pump inhibitors (FDA Drug Safety Communication, 2011, March 2):[10]

> *[3-2-2011] The U.S. Food and Drug Administration (FDA) is informing the public that prescription proton pump inhibitor (PPI) drugs may cause low serum magnesium levels (hypomagnesemia) if taken for prolonged periods of time (in most cases, longer than one year). In approximately one-quarter of the cases reviewed, magnesium supplementation alone did not improve low serum magnesium levels and the PPI had to be discontinued.*

Note the last sentence in the quote, which has been emphasized here with bold print for the purposes of this discussion. This is a very, very serious health issue, to say the least, not only from a PC risk standpoint, but because magnesium is a vital electrolyte, An adequate supply is necessary for the normal performance of many critical chemical and neurological processes that go on continuously in the body.

Our paleo ancestors didn't drink coffee or alcohol, and they didn't use medications.

While it's almost certain that they may have used a selection of natural remedies for various ailments, it's not likely that they used any treatments that depleted magnesium. So our digestive system evolved without any allowance for magnesium-depleting foods, beverages, or medications.

This important difference is probably the main reason why magnesium deficiency is so common these days. Many authorities claim that magnesium and other minerals have been severely depleted from soils used for food production, and surely there is some truth to this.

But it's likely that the main problem can be found in the way that so many aspects of our modern lifestyle deplete the magnesium in our diet. Food processing often results in reduced magnesium content. Modern humans put far too many things into their bodies that did not exist when the human digestive system was evolving over millions of years, and the combined effect of all these items is stealing our magnesium.

One of the many benefits of magnesium supplementation is eliminating leg or foot cramps.

Magnesium also resolves so-called restless leg syndrome. If you have these symptoms you very likely have a magnesium deficiency and the symptoms should begin to resolve soon after you begin supplementing with an adequate amount of magnesium. It's true that a deficiency of other electrolytes can also cause leg or foot cramps, but the most common electrolyte deficiency by far appears to be magnesium deficiency.

Do you crave chocolate?

Chocolate is a good source of magnesium. Medical statistics show that those who crave chocolate are typically magnesium deficient.

There are many other symptoms of magnesium deficiency.

Obviously not everyone who is magnesium deficient has all of these symptoms, and some symptoms may go unnoticed or they may be attributed to some other cause, but all of these are known to be associated with magnesium deficiency. And taking an adequate magnesium supplement should resolve the symptoms.

Symptoms can include (but are not limited to) muscle weakness, muscle twitches, pain, tremors, tingling or numbness in hands or feet, low energy, fatigue, unexplained weight loss, insomnia, heart palpitations or tachycardia (high heart rate), irritability , profuse sweating, shortness of breath or the inability to draw a deep breath, hypertension or erratic blood pressure, migraines, brittle nails, slow nail growth, recurring skin or urinary tract infections, recurring vaginal yeast infections, brain fog, depression, constipation, foul body odor, frequent urination, urination urgency, kidney stones, kidney disease, dry mouth, excessive thirst, dry itchy skin, tooth decay, osteoporosis, confusion, irritability, anxiety, panic attacks, apathy, anorexia, memory problems, and compromised learning ability (University of Maryland Medical Center, n.d., Sircus, 2009, December 8, Schachter, 1996).[11,12,13] Note that some of these symptoms are the same symptoms seen with diabetes because (as we shall see on pages 25–26 in chapter 3) magnesium deficiency causes insulin resistance and reduced insulin production by the pancreas.

In cases of severe magnesium deficiency, breathing problems can develop.

Breathing problems associated with magnesium deficiency are somewhat unique. Because breathing is normally automatically controlled by the autonomic nervous system, whenever a breathing issue occurs because of an episode of acute magnesium deficiency, the patient will become very aware of her or his breathing. Almost every breath will become a conscious effort. There will be an urge to take a deep breath, but on most attempts the patient will be unable to take a deep breath. Because theses episodes often occur late at night, in some situations patients will wonder if they woke up because their body forgot to breathe, and they will be afraid to go back to sleep for fear of not awakening the next time it happens.

Breathing can even seem labored, almost like an asthma attack except that there will be no wheezing. When patients ask their doctors for an explanation of what is wrong with them to cause such symptoms, the response may be a blank stare, because physicians are typically not properly trained to recognize magnesium deficiency symptoms, so this problem is not likely to even be on their radar.

Doctors will sometimes diagnose the condition as hyperventilation disorder. But the root cause is magnesium deficiency. The mechanism by which this occurs appears to be associated with compromised nerve function and weakened muscle response in the diaphragm, resulting in reduced breathing capacity. This observation is supported by research showing that children who are magnesium deficient tend to have reduced lung function (Gilliland, Berhane, Li, Kim, & Margolis, 2002).[14] But because of this apparent omission in medical school training, if patients don't figure out the cause of the problem themselves, it may never be resolved.

Magnesium deficiency can cause seizures.

Case studies suggest that in some cases chronic magnesium deficiency can eventually lead to epileptic seizures (Nuytten, Van Hees, Meulemans, & Carton, 1991).[15] Furthermore, research studies have shown that people who have epilepsy tend to have lower magnesium levels than people who do not have the condition (Yuen, & Sander, 2012).[16] These researchers have suggested that magnesium supplementation might be successfully used to reduce epileptic seizures.

Another tipoff of a long-term magnesium deficiency is brittle nails.

Many people mistakenly believe that brittle nails are caused by a calcium deficiency, but this is not the case. Calcium utilization is regulated by magnesium and vitamin D. Virtually everyone has plenty of calcium in their diet. So when issues that appear to be associated with calcium deficiency appear (such as osteoporosis, for example), it's time to look for a vitamin D or magnesium deficiency, or both. Chronic magnesium deficiency can definitely cause brittle nails and slow nail growth if the deficiency is moderate to severe.

Magnesium deficiency can be caused by genetics.

Some people are unable to absorb magnesium as well as others (Mauskop, & Varughese, 2012). And various other issues can either compromise the absorption of magnesium or cause it to be wasted by the renal system. As Galland (1991–1992) pointed out, even psychological stress can cause magnesium to be wasted by the kidneys, and this can result in a magnesium deficiency.[17]

How magnesium supplements are taken can affect the amount absorbed.

Taking larger doses of magnesium at one time can result in wasted magnesium because as the blood level increases, the absorption rate tends to decline. So dividing the total daily dose into several smaller amounts taken at various times during the day, such as at mealtimes, can help to improve the total amount absorbed.

Could a chronic magnesium deficiency lead to the development of type 2 diabetes?

As we will see in the next chapter, it's well known that magnesium deficiency is correlated with insulin resistance, and it's a medical fact that many people who have type 2 diabetes have low blood magnesium levels. This connection is very likely the reason why diabetes is also closely associated with pancreatic cancer. Diabetes is listed in this book as a separate risk for the development of pancreatic cancer, but bear in mind that magnesium deficiency might possibly be the primary reason why diabetes is associated with PC.

But why does taking a magnesium supplement reduce the risk of developing pancreatic cancer?

For one thing, magnesium is a vital electrolyte. So when it becomes deficient, some of the many normal body processes that depend on it may not be able to proceed normally, and this can have adverse consequences if it occurs on a regular basis. For example, a magnesium deficiency obviously has a potent effect on the pancreas because (again, as we shall see in the next chapter) it causes the pancreas to produce less insulin. Magnesium is also known to have anti-inflammatory properties.

This observation is pure speculation, but there is a very good chance that the reason why magnesium helps to prevent PC may be due to this anti-inflammatory characteristic. C-reactive protein is commonly used as a way to measure the level of inflammation in the body. Research shows that taking a magnesium supplement reduces C-reactive protein levels.

One study based on sample data from the National Health and Nutrition Examination Survey that covered the years 1999–2002 showed that among U. S. adults who were not taking a magnesium supplement, only

21.9 % met or exceeded the RDA for magnesium (King, Mainous, Geesey, Egan, & Rehman, 2006).[18] ;These researchers concluded that people whose total daily magnesium intake was less than the RDA were approximately 40 % more likely to have an elevated C-reactive protein level.

And here's something else to remember about magnesium.

There is evidence that many (probably most) cases of depression may be due to magnesium deficiency. Eby & Eby (2006) published case studies to show that magnesium supplementation often brings rapid recovery of depression symptoms, in addition to resolving many other health issues.[19] It's not likely that additional research based on dedicated, random controlled trials will be pursued to investigate this line of treatment however, because most research is funded by the big pharmaceutical companies and they are making far too much money developing new, ridiculously expensive medications to treat anxiety and depression. It would be counterproductive for them to spend money on research that might conclude that magnesium supplementation could be used to treat or prevent depression, as that would surely reduce the sales of many drugs.

Magnesium is not just another nutrient.

As we have already discussed in this chapter, magnesium is an electrolyte that's absolutely essential for the completion of many essential processes required continually by many of the systems that allow the human body to function normally. So it shouldn't come as a surprise that a chronic magnesium deficiency may be an accident waiting to happen. And this is why when you read chapter 11, you will clearly understand that a chronic magnesium deficiency was almost surely the initial problem that lead to other dietary issues and then combined with those issues to eventually lead to the death of Steve Jobs.

Summary

Most people living in developed countries today are magnesium deficient. Many things are known to deplete magnesium, including many medications, digestive system issues, and certain foods and drinks including coffee and alcohol. Regardless of how much magnesium might be in one's diet, published, peer-reviewed medical research shows that those who do not take a magnesium supplement have approximately twice the risk of developing pancreatic cancer as those who take a magnesium supplement that meets or exceeds the recommended RDA. And as a bonus, taking a magnesium supplement provides many other health benefits for most people.

Chapter 3

Diabetes Is Strongly Associated With Pancreatic Cancer

Because of the strong association, it's especially important for diabetes patients to take precautions to minimize their risks.

While it's not clear whether diabetes always precedes pancreatic cancer or pancreatic cancer causes diabetes, research published by Batabyal, Vander Hoorn, Christophi, and Nikfarjam (2014) makes it disturbingly clear that having diabetes doubles the risk of PC.[20]

Note that their study shows that in some cases the development of diabetes may be a symptom of PC.

This is suggested by the fact that diabetes patients in the study were 7 times as likely to be diagnosed with PC during the first year after they were diagnosed with diabetes, compared with someone who did not have diabetes. That's an extremely high correlation.

An earlier group of researchers had found that pancreatic cancer patients have either glucose intolerance or "frank diabetes" in approximately 80 % of cases (Wang, Herrington, Larsson, & Permert, 2003).[21] "Frank diabetes" is simply a medical term used to describe the stage of the disease at which the use of medications becomes necessary. Again, note that this is a very high correlation.

As evidence that pancreatic cancer causes diabetes, the researchers pointed out that in most cases where diabetes is associated with PC, the diabetes is either diagnosed at the same time as the cancer, or during a 2-year period immediately preceding the PC diagnosis (Gullo, Pezzilli, Morselli-Labate, & the Italian Pancreatic Cancer Study Group, 1994).[22] This suggests that the diabetes markers are triggered by the development of the cancer and furthermore, maybe these markers should be interpreted as possible early warning signs of PC.

Also, in 71 % of cases the patient's glucose intolerance is unknown prior to the PC diagnosis (Schwarts, Zeidler, Moossa, Kuku, & Rubenstein, 1978).[23] This also supports the suggestion that these markers may be early warning signs of PC.

It's also worth noting that when PC patients undergo surgery to remove the tumor, their insulin resistance and diabetes symptoms in general tend to significantly improve within several months following the surgery (Permert et al., 1993).[24] Obviously that suggests that the symptoms were almost surely caused by the tumor in the first place.

But researchers have also concluded that diabetes can lead to the development of pancreatic cancer (Everhart & Wright, 1995).[25] Their data suggest that diabetes may roughly double the odds of developing PC for at least 5 years following a diagnosis (of diabetes). But after 5 years have passed, the research results from various studies show conflicting results, so it's unclear whether the increased risk persists past about 5 years or gradually fades away.

However, whether or not the risk cited by that research lasts longer than 5 years may be a moot point because in chapter 11 of this book we will learn that PC typically takes much longer than 5 years to develop before it is likely to reach a stage at which it can be diagnosed. That's a confounding factor for the conclusion reached by Everhart and Wright (1995), and therefore it invalidates their conclusion because any case of pancreatic cancer diagnosed within 5 years after a diagnosis of diabetes almost surely existed before diabetes was diagnosed.

But this leads us to the magnesium connection again.

As mentioned in the previous chapter, magnesium deficiency plays an important role in the development of insulin resistance and type 2 diabetes. Researchers have shown that both hypertension and type 2 diabetes involve low intracellular magnesium levels (Takaya, Higashino, & Kobayashi, 2004).[26] In the research article cited, Takaya, Higashino, and Kobayashi (2004) concluded that because magnesium is necessary for the proper utilization of glucose, and it's also used for insulin signaling, an intracellular magnesium deficiency may alter glucose availability and contribute to the development of insulin resistance.

Magnesium and insulin are co-dependent.

One cannot function properly without the other. And this is a 2-way street in many regards. Not only does a magnesium deficiency cause insulin resistance in the cells of the body, and reduced insulin production by the pancreas, but there is a reciprocal effect. Insulin is responsible for the transport of nutrients to locations where they can either be immediately utilized or stored for future use. When the availability and effectiveness of insulin is compromised, extra magnesium in the blood cannot be properly stored, so most of it may be wasted, instead (Sircus, 2009).[27]

This can dramatically increase the odds that diabetes patients may develop a magnesium deficiency. And of course as the magnesium deficiency becomes worse, insulin resistance may increase and insulin production by the pancreas may decline even further.

But even stronger evidence of the association between magnesium deficiency and diabetes has been found by researchers. Research published by Hruby et al. (2014) found that higher magnesium intake reduces the risk of insulin resistance and the risk of progression from a prediabetic condition to diabetes.[28] In that study, people who had the highest magnesium intake had only about half the risk (53 %) of metabolic interference or diabetes development compared with those who had the lowest magnesium intake. This information is especially important for those who have been told by their physicians that their blood test results indicate that they are at a stage known as prediabetes.

Gastroparesis (slow stomach emptying) is a common problem with diabetes.

It's a serious problem for almost a third of diabetes patients because it can cause nausea, acid reflux, and other problems, and doctors seem flummoxed by this issue. But it is likely that researchers will some day show that gastroparesis is typically caused by magnesium deficiency. Muscles cannot perform properly without adequate magnesium. They cannot relax, and they tend to spasm and develop tremors.

The pyloric sphincter is located between the stomach and the first segment of the small intestine (known as the duodenum). The pyloric sphincter is regulated by the enteric nervous system to allow chyme (partially digested food) to flow from the stomach into the small intestine as the stomach completes it's part of the digestive process. The adverse effects of magnesium deficiency on the central nervous system are well known and there's no obvious reason not to attribute the same association to the enteric nervous system (Langley, & Mann, 1991).[29] The enteric nervous system, sometimes called the second brain, controls the digestive system and correlates information between the digestive system and the brain.

This particular observation does not seem to have been explored by medical researchers, so there is no published medical proof of this theory, but it seems apparent that a magnesium deficiency would be very likely to interfere with the proper functioning of the pyloric sphincter. And compromised functioning could prevent it from allowing the stomach to empty properly as chyme is ready to be passed into the small intestine. Chyme that remains in the stomach too long tends to ferment in the warm, moist environment, producing gas and pressure that can cause nausea.

This can also cause acid reflux and gastroesophageal reflux disease (GERD) because if the pyloric sphincter cannot function properly because of a magnesium deficiency, then the lower esophageal sphincter between the esophagus and the stomach probably will not function well enough to prevent acid reflux, either. And we already know that diabetes is closely associated with magnesium deficiency. Therefore, to resolve a gastroparesis problem, most diabetes patients probably simply need magnesium, rather than the drugs that most doctors prescribe to treat the problem.

Is there a difference in the PC risks associated with type 1 or type 2 diabetes?

A few studies have indicated that an increased risk of PC is not associated with type I diabetes (Hjalgrim et al., 1997).[30] But it appears that most studies have not distinguished between the 2 types. Statistically, it's likely that only a relatively small percentage of type I cases are involved in these studies because roughly 90 % of total diabetes cases are type 2.

The message is clear, however.

If a patient's doctor is not already in the process of cautiously ruling out pancreatic cancer, anyone who has recently been diagnosed with diabetes, would be very prudent to encourage their doctors to rule it out as soon as possible, just to be on the safe side. The increased risk declines as the years pass, but for the first 5–10 years after a type 2 diabetes diagnosis, increased vigilance can safe lives by catching PC early enough (if it is present) that it may be treatable.

There can be certain clues that may add urgency to the need to rule out PC when type 2 diabetes is diagnosed. For example, type 2 diabetes usually causes an increased appetite and it does not cause weight loss. Therefore a loss of appetite or loss of weight along with a recent diagnosis of type 2 diabetes would be a huge red flag regarding PC risk.

It's well known that reducing the risk of developing diabetes boils down to a matter of lifestyle choices. For example, research even suggests that something as simple as eating home-cooked meals can reduce the risk of developing Type 2 diabetes (Zong, Eisenberg, Hu, & Sun, 2016).[31] Nutrition issues are often blamed on the increasing popularity of eating more meals away from home , much of which falls into the so-called "fast food" category. It's claimed that this trend increases the risk of poor nutrition habits, resulting in increased risk of health problems such as type 2 diabetes (ScienceDaily, 2016, July 5).[32]

But as Zong, Eisenbert, Hu, & Sun (2016) noted:

> *The main limitations of our study were that it lacked assessments on individual foods constituting the MPAH and that the findings were limited to health professionals with a relatively homogeneous socioeconomic status.*

Those are major limitations and they raise some serious questions about whether or not the results might actually be valid for the general population. For one thing, there are no studies verifying that health professionals tend to have the same dietary habits as the general population. Do they practice what they preach when they sit down to eat? Or do they leave their professional advice at the office?

But there's an even broader concern about the results of the study.

There's a very good possibility that confounding issues in the study such as the widespread use of partially hydrogenated oils (aka trans fats) in the fast food industry during the years covered by that study may have skewed the results. Doesn't it seem likely that meals prepared at home during those years may have contained less trans fats, and this could have been responsible for the health advantages of eating at home found by the study?

But even if these reservations about the study results should turn out to be true, the implications regarding the risk of developing PC should still be valid That is, eating meals prepared at home should decrease the risk of developing PC by virtue of decreasing the risk of type 2 diabetes.

Summary

Diabetes is closely associated with pancreatic cancer, and in some cases diabetes may be a symptom of pancreatic cancer. But because diabetes is also closely associated with magnesium deficiency, and it's known that most pancreatic cancer patients have a magnesium deficiency, it's possible that the magnesium deficiency connection may be the primary reason for the association of diabetes with pancreatic cancer.

Chapter 4

Vitamin D Deficiency and Pancreatic Cancer

Research shows that pancreatic cancer rates are higher in countries that have lower levels of ultraviolet B irradiation.

A derivative of cholesterol, 7-dehydrocholesterol is present on the surface of the skin, and the action of ultraviolet B irradiation converts it into vitamin D3. For decades, mainstream medicine has largely misunderstood many aspects of the role of cholesterol in the human body. This has resulted in widespread inappropriate efforts to suppress cholesterol levels in broad categories of people who are not at risk of cardiovascular events, despite published research studies showing that lowering cholesterol levels does not improve longevity, nor does lowering cholesterol levels reduce cardiovascular risks for the general population (Ramsden et al., 2016).[33]

There are 2 common forms of vitamin D available as supplements, D2 and D3. Vitamin D2 is the form most often prescribed by physicians to treat vitamin D deficiency, and vitamin D3 is the form produced by our skin when exposed to sunlight. Vitamin D3 seems to be more effective for boosting blood vitamin D levels, and it is the type most often offered in over-the-counter vitamin D supplements.

Researchers have discovered that roughly 80 % of one's cholesterol level is determined by genetics, so obviously diet can only have a relatively minor effect (Thompson, 2015).[34] And contrary to the guidelines currently followed by most health "experts", these studies have also demonstrated that raising HDL cholesterol levels does not provide any mortality risk benefits (Keene, Price, Shun-Shin, & Francis, 2014).[35]

This suggests that most of the medical advice we have received about cholesterol during our lifetimes has been incorrect.

The implications of this research contradict and pretty much nullify much of the conventional wisdom that was previously used as a basis for establishing medical policies regarding cholesterol levels and how they affect (or do not effect) the health of most individuals in the general population. These data demand that the tests currently being used to assess patient cardiovascular health must be reevaluated and a completely revised approach be developed regarding the ways that mainstream medical practitioners apply this information.

But in the meantime, this misguided, decades-long campaign designed to suppress cholesterol levels, plus the widespread use of sunscreen products, has resulted in an epidemic of vitamin D deficiency. The main problem with the existing recommendations is that suppressing cholesterol levels also suppresses the production of vitamin D in the skin. Whether this policy has had a significant adverse effect on the overall health of the general population is yet to be proven, but surely it has contributed to the trend toward inadequate vitamin D levels for many, many people. This limits the effectiveness of the immune system and puts many people at an increased risk of many health issues, including cancer. Compared with their grandparents and great-grandparents, most people today only produce a fraction of the vitamin D that their forebears produced.

Vitamin D deficiency is so common that the FDA has recently decided to add vitamin D to the labeling requirements for all processed foods sold in the U. S.[36]

This officially acknowledges the fact that most Americans are not getting enough vitamin D. Our grandparents and great grandparents got most of their vitamin D from the sun. But today, the combination of air conditioning and the misguided cholesterol and sunscreen policies described in the previous paragraphs has led to a health crisis of sorts where vitamin D deficiency is the rule.

Many health advisors (who should know better) promote the illusion that any deficits caused by lower vitamin D production in the skin can be easily made up from the diet. But in the real world that option typically does not even come close to supplying enough vitamin D to make up for the deficit. As pointed out by the Vitamin D Council, relying on diet sources of vitamin D to make up for deficiencies is usually wishful thinking.[37] And the problem is compounded by official (from the government's Institute of Medicine) published RDA guidelines that have been contradicted by published research and shown to be woefully inadequate for preventing most diseases (Persky, 2013, pp. 78–88).

Vitamin D is utilized by the body when the active form of vitamin D binds to Vitamin D receptors (VDRs) in tissues. VDRs are present in both normal cells and in cancer cells. Albrechtsson et al. (2003) found that VDRs were present in all of the different types of pancreatic cancer cells analyzed in their study.[38] And in 6 types of pancreatic cancer, more than 3 times as many VDRs were present than can be typically found in normal pancreatic cells. That makes these cancer strains particularly vulnerable to vitamin D.

Furthermore, the researchers found that relatively high doses of a synthetic form of vitamin D3 could be used to decrease the number of pancreatic cancer cells. And this finding held true for all of the types of PC cells that were studied. Because this clearly shows that vitamin D is capable of destroying pancreatic cancer cells, this strongly suggests that pancreatic cancer may be associated with vitamin D deficiency.

Unfortunately, attempts to prove that observation have met with mixed results. Some studies have shown that high blood vitamin D levels are associated with low PC risk. But other studies have not shown that association.

It's well known that the residents of countries that have lower levels of ultraviolet B (UVB) irradiation tend to have lower blood levels of vitamin D. At least 1 study has shown that in countries with low UVB radiation levels, residents are approximately 6 times as likely to develop PC, compared with the residents of countries that have relatively high UVB levels (Garlanda, Cuomob, Gorhama, Zenga, & Mohra, 2016).[39] Thus countries that have more cloud cover or anything else that limits UVB exposure tend to have significantly higher rates of PC. And this correlates with well known relationships between sun exposure and vitamin D levels.

The effects of UVB exposure and vitamin D are associated with many cancers, not just pancreatic cancer. In a recently-published study (Fleischer, & Fleischer, 2016) the authors made this observation:[40]

> *We found that cancer incidence for all invasive cancers and for 11 of 22 leading cancers significantly decreased with increased solar radiation.*

> *Cancer mortality for all invasive cancers was not significantly associated with solar radiation, but for 7 of 22 leading cancers, including cancers of the uterus, leukemias, lung, ovary, and urinary bladder, increased solar radiation predicted decreased mortality.*

Without adequate vitamin D, the immune system cannot function properly to safeguard the body's health as it was designed to do. Vulnerability to disease increases significantly as blood levels of vitamin D drop. Therefore it is advisable to occasionally have one's vitamin D level checked to make sure that it is well up in the adequate (not merely sufficient) range. If test results are not available, the Vitamin D Council suggests that a safe daily supplement for most adults is approximately 5,000 IU of vitamin D3 (Cannell, 2013).[41]

Interestingly, very recently published research comparing mortality risks with blood levels of vitamin D shows that pancreatic cancer patients who had higher vitamin D serum levels were much more likely to survive than those who had lower vitamin D levels (Yuan et al., 2016).[42] In the study, blood vitamin D levels (25[OH]D levels) above 30 ng/mL were considered to be sufficient, levels below 20 ng/mL were considered to be insufficient, and those in between (20–30 ng/mL) were listed as "relative insufficiency". Approximately 33 % of the 493 patients in the study were found to be vitamin D insufficient. Yuan et al. (2016) showed that patients with relative insufficiency were found to have 79 % of the mortality risk of the patients who had insufficient vitamin D levels, and patients who had sufficient blood levels of vitamin D were found to have only 66 % of the mortality risk of those patients who had insufficient vitamin D levels.

When only patients whose blood had been tested within 5 years of diagnosis were considered, those who had a blood vitamin D level equal to or above 30 ng/mL had only 58 % of the mortality risk of those whose blood vitamin D level was below 20 ng/mL. In other words, it only took a 10 ng/mL increase in blood vitamin D levels to cut the risk of mortality almost in half.

Sadly, no comparisons were made for higher vitamin D levels, possibly because so few patients with higher vitamin D levels ever develop pancreatic cancer. Whether that speculation is true or not, clearly, higher vitamin D levels significantly improve the survival rates associated with pancreatic cancer.

Summary

The association of vitamin D deficiency with many types of cancer is well documented. Research has shown that people who live in the countries of the world that have the lowest levels of UVB radiation have approximately 6 times the risk of developing pancreatic cancer compared with those living in countries where the highest levels of UVB radiation is available. That strongly suggests that vitamin D deficiency may be associated with an increased risk of developing pancreatic cancer.

Published research also shows that lower blood vitamin D levels are associated with higher mortality rates of pancreatic cancer. Patients who have vitamin D blood levels generally considered to be insufficient (below 20 ng/mL) may have almost double the mortality risk of those who have sufficient vitamin D levels (above 30 ng/mL).

Chapter 5

Oral Bacteria and Pancreatic Cancer

The bacteria that live in our mouth may affect our risk of developing the disease.

Research published in 2013 shows that one of the common species of bacteria responsible for causing gum disease, Porphyromonas gingivalis, thrives by defeating the human immune system (Gaddis, Maynard, Weaver, Michalek, & Katz, 2013).[43] It manages to pull off this trick by promoting the production of an anti-inflammatory agent, Interleukin-10 (IL-10). Normally the immune system would send out T cells to destroy such bacteria and they would take care of the problem. But the presence of IL-10 prevents T cells from doing their job. So the bacteria are able to thrive under the radar of the immune system.

Why is this a concern in a book about pancreatic cancer? Because over half of Americans develop periodontal disease after they pass the age of 50. And because P. gingivalis is able to evade the human immune system, gum disease and the complicating infections that can be associated with it tend to be extremely difficult to treat effectively. Without any help from the immune system, eradication can prove to be quite a challenge. This allows the bacterial infections to be incredibly persistent. In other words, they can become established as a chronic condition.

8 Ways to Prevent Pancreatic Cancer

The significance of this threat becomes obvious in view of a research discovery published in 2016 that connects bacteria responsible for periodontal disease with the risk of developing pancreatic cancer. Researchers found that there is a 59 % increased risk of developing pancreatic cancer associated with P. gingivalis and at least a 50 % increased risk of developing PC associated with Aggregatibacter actinomycetemcomitans (Scutti, 2016, Garchitorena, 2016).[44,45]

Obviously much research remains to be done to identify the exact details of how these bacteria manage to increase the risk of developing PC, but the evidence suggests that they may migrate to the pancreas. Because they (at least this has been verified for P. gingivalis) can escape detection by the immune system, if they were to establish an infection in the pancreas, they would have all the time needed to create an environment suitable for the development of cancer.

Other researchers have verified, for example, that the bacterium A. actinomycetemcomitans is capable of migrating from lesions in the mouth to other organs and establishing infections there (Wang et al., 2010).[46] Wang et al. (2010) cited examples involving infective endocarditis (infections involving the heart), osteonecrosis (death of bone tissue usually due to reduced blood flow), pneumonia (lungs), and lesions in the chest wall. So clearly, these bacteria are capable of causing very serious problems in areas other than the gums.

Summary
Certain bacteria commonly associated with gum disease have been shown to be associated with a significantly increased risk of pancreatic cancer.

Chapter 6

Poultry and Pancreatic Cancer

An unidentified issue with chickens causes them to be closely associated with pancreatic cancer.

Between the years of 1992 and 2000, a huge study involving the collection and analysis of data on almost half a million people in 10 European countries was begun. The study is known as the European Prospective Investigation into Cancer and Nutrition (EPIC). As the data have been analyzed, some interesting observations have been noted (Rohrmann et al., 2013).[47]

The study noted that by 2008, 865 cases of pancreatic cancer were recorded that were of nonendocrine origin. Roughly 95 % of pancreatic cancer tumors are classified as nonendocrine. Nonendocrine tumors develop much more aggressively than neuroendocrine tumors.

But some of the dietary association results were surprising.

The study showed that the consumption of red meat for example, and processed meat, had no association with an increased risk of pancreatic cancer. Clearly this contradicts the World Cancer Research Fund's claim that the consumption of red meat or processed meat may increase the risk of developing pancreatic cancer. And as expected, no increased risk was found among those who regularly ate fish.

But the most surprising discovery appears to be the association between the consumption of poultry and the risk of developing pancreatic cancer.

Poultry consumption was definitely associated with a significantly increased risk of PC. No one knows why this association might exist, but there is no apparent reason to dispute the data. The data show a 72 % increased risk of PC for every 50 grams (1.7637 ounces) of poultry in the average daily diet. That implies, for example, that someone who eats approximately 8 ounces of poultry daily would have more than triple the risk (327 %) of developing pancreatic cancer compared with someone who does not eat poultry.

This finding is especially ironic in view of the decades-long advertising claims promoting chicken as a safer alternative to red meat. Surely this persuaded many people to eat much more chicken than they would have were it not for the advertising claims.

Incidentally, a similar study of the data in the EPIC project revealed that vegetarians in the study had a 39 % increased risk of developing colon cancer when compared with meat eaters (Key et al., 2009).[48] Again, this contradicts conventional thinking and promotional claims.

But more than that, this raises an interesting question. The study shows that compared with eating red meat, eating poultry significantly increases the risk of developing pancreatic cancer, and the data show that avoiding red meat (by following a vegetarian diet) increases the risk of colon cancer. Despite all the apparently misguided propaganda against the consumption of red meat for all these years, could red meat in the diet offer some degree of protection against pancreatic and other types of cancer? After all, this is a huge study involving hundreds of thousands of people over a period of many, many years. The apparent distortion of reality that was associated with the campaign against red meat, whether intentional or accidental, may go down in history as a prime example of how paid lobbyists, well-funded advertising campaigns, and inappropriate government support can distort the truth to create and perpetuate false health claims that can adversely affect the health of many, many people in the general population.

But just working with poultry and animals destined for slaughter appears to increase the risk of developing pancreatic cancer, especially for certain people who work in poultry production and processing. A study report published by Felini et al. (2011) showed that workers who slaughter poultry were 8.9 times as likely to develop PC as someone in the general population.[49] The increased risk of developing PC was 3.6 for workers whose job involved merely catching live chickens.

But poultry workers also have a significantly increased risk of liver cancer.

While the cause of the increased risk of PC and liver cancer has never been proven, it's suspected that the oncogenic viruses carried by chickens (and many other animals) may be responsible. Oncogenic viruses include any viruses capable of creating tumors, including herpesviruses, papillomaviruses, polyomaviruses, poxviruses, and retroviruses. The risk of developing liver cancer by workers who slaughtered chickens was found to be 9.1 times the risk for controls (Felini et al., 2011).

Just working on a pig farm at any time in their life tripled the risk of developing PC for the people in that study. And workers who slaughtered animals in the meat processing industry had an increased PC risk of 4.8.

Interestingly, the same study (Felini et al., 2011) showed that a vaccination for yellow fever increased the risk of developing liver cancer (but not PC) to 8.7 times that of controls, and a typhoid vaccination increased the risk of liver cancer to 6.3 times the rate for controls.

The report speculated that possibly the viruses associated with poultry might play a role in the increased risks for the development of pancreatic cancer. But the fact that workers who slaughtered other animals had a 400 % PC risk increase suggests that close contact with the body fluids of birds and animals in general may increase the risk of pancreatic cancer. Obviously more research is needed.

Previous studies have been undertaken to assess the human risks associated with working around poultry. Chickens and turkeys are hosts to many viruses that cause cancer (in poultry) (Netto & Johnson, 2003).[50] Research by Netto and Johnson (2003) shows that not only is there a significant risk associated with working around poultry, but poultry products can also pose risks. This research project investigated mortality in a group of 7,700 members of a local poultry union in the state of Missouri between the years of 1969—1990.

The study found statistically significant (relatively high) rates of respiratory disease, senility, accidents, and various adverse events But because these subjects were typically relatively young, mortality rates at the end of the study were low, making it difficult to assign statistical significance to the findings regarding cancer cases.

While public exposure to any possible poultry risks are generally more limited than poultry workers, as the research report points out, the risks go far beyond contact with, and the consumption of poultry meat and eggs. Most vaccines are produced in the embryo cells in eggs. As noted by Johnson (1994), certain avian viruses are very common in poultry flocks and they are known to cause cancer in poultry.[51] The various strains of the avian leukosis/sarcoma group (ALSV) are examples.

In 1999, Tsang et al. reported that all of the measles and mumps vaccines in use in the United States (at the time of the report) were contaminated with ALSV.[52] But they also reported that all of the blood samples taken from 33 children following vaccination showed no evidence of the virus. 33 is a very small number on which to base meaningful statistics, but hopefully that will continue to be the case.

In the same year (1999) Pham et al. found that at least 14 % of the chicken egg samples taken from 20 randomly-selected New Orleans retail stores were contaminated with avian leukosis retroviruses.[53] Obviously, exposure to sources of the viruses would be difficult to avoid for most people today. Still, remember that the results of the 2013 study mentioned at the start of this chapter only applied to people who ate poultry flesh regularly. Any other risks would be in addition to that.

Summary

According to research, poultry carry unidentified threats to human health that significantly increase the risk of developing pancreatic cancer (and other issues). Eating poultry products increases this risk, and the increase in risk may possibly extend to eggs and even vaccines.

The increased risk is especially significant for some occupations associated with raising, handling, and slaughtering animals for food. And work that involves the slaughter of poultry, has been found to be associated with an exceptionally large increase in the risk of PC. In addition, some of these work categories appear to be associated with an abnormally-high risk of liver cancer. While the cause of these large risk increases is still unproven, it's suspected that oncogenic viruses in poultry and other animals may be responsible.

Chapter 7

Soy and Pancreatic Cancer

Soy is a relatively recent addition to the so-called Western diet — it was only introduced slightly over half a century ago.

More than 3 decades ago, researchers Guinness, Morgan, and Wormsley (1984) discovered that if rats were fed raw soybean flour for longer than a year, approximately 10 % of them would develop pancreatic cancer.[54] But even more importantly, the soy flour made the rats vulnerable to exposures to tiny amounts of carcinogens that would normally be too weak to initiate a pancreatic cancer tumor.

> *If the raw soya flour-containing diets are fed for more than a year, about 10% of the animals develop pancreatic cancer. In addition, feeding raw soya flour markedly potentiates the action of even subthreshold amounts of pancreatic carcinogens. The raw soya flour therefore acts as a potent promoter, as well as a weak carcinogen. (p. 205)*

Guiness, Morgan, and Wormsley (1984) also strongly encouraged additional research to either verify or rule out similar effects on humans, but it's not clear from the literature that this has ever been done.

> *It is not known whether the human pancreas responds to dietary trypsin inhibitors in a manner similar to the rat. However, in view of*

the use of soya-based products in human nutrition--especially in infant foods--we urge that the effect of all soya-based products intended for human use be tested on the rat pancreas in long-term feeding studies, combined with subthreshold doses of azaserine to highlight any promoting activity of the product. (p. 205)

Unless they are fermented first, soybeans are very difficult for humans to digest. In Japan, for centuries certain species of soybeans have been traditionally fermented before using them for human consumption. But not only are soybeans not fermented before use in most other countries, (including the U. S.), but the varieties of soybeans grown are different from those grown in Japan.

Digestion of soy requires protease enzyme, which is produced by the pancreas. But unfortunately soybeans contain protease inhibitors that prevent the protease enzyme from working properly (Daniel, n.d.).[55] As a result, the pancreas has to work much harder to produce additional protease enzyme. Research shows that over time, if soy is a regular part of the diet, this leads to an increase in the number of pancreatic cells and an increase in the size of those cells.

From a cellular histology viewpoint, this amounts to hyperplasia and hypertrophy of pancreatic cells.

This is concerning because these cellular changes are often seen with the development of malignancy. As Daniel (n.d.) points out, continued ingestion of soy can lead to swelling of the pancreas and digestive distress, and this can be especially problematic for young people as a result of the negative effects on growth.

The increase in PC fatalities seems to correlate with the use of soybeans in this country.

Certain varieties of soybeans (not grown in the U. S.) have been part of the human diet in Japan and other Asian countries for hundreds and in some cases thousands of years. But before the 1940s, the only significant use of soybeans in the U. S. was for livestock forage and green fertilizer to be plowed into the soil. Because soybeans are a legume, they are nitrogen-fixing, and therefore they can be used to capture and add nitrogen fertilizer to the soil. During the 1940s, farmers began to harvest the beans and feed them to livestock, and after that, soybean production began to expand rapidly during the '50s, '60s, and '70s.

At some point during the 1980s, food manufacturers "discovered" that soybeans were a cheap source of protein that could be used in a lot of foods and this led to a significant increase in the amount of soy in the American diet. In 1991, the National Soybean Checkoff (which amounted to a government-enforced tax on soybeans at the farm level, with the proceeds used to promote the sales of soybean-based products) went into effect. This resulted in a huge increase in the use of soybeans in food, pharmaceuticals, cosmetics, and many other consumer products.

This surge in soybean use for human food in the U. S. also coincides with the shift to earlier puberty in children (especially in females), presumably because of the estrogen-like effects of isoflavones in soybeans (Adgent et al., 2012, Kim, Kim, Huh, Kim, & Joung, 2011).[56,57] If soy can influence the age of puberty, then it doesn't take much of a stretch of the imagination to realize that it can probably affect other body functions that are regulated by hormones. Once hormone production is altered somewhere in the body there can be a domino effect as altered hormone production in one organ causes altered hormone production in organs that are regulated by the hormones produced by the first organ. The end results can be impossible to predict.

And soy is another PC-associated risk that can be linked back to magnesium deficiency.[58] Soy has a high phytic acid content, which implies that it interferes with the absorption of important minerals such as calcium, copper, iron, magnesium, and zinc. And as pointed out by Miller (2013), four very undesirable substances are found in soybeans — hemagglutinin, nitrites, soy protein isolates, and goitrogens.

Hemagglutinin causes red blood cells to clump together. Obviously that characteristic can cause unanticipated clotting problems. The carcinogenic (cancer-causing) properties of nitrites are well known. Soy protein isolates tend to contain trypsin inhibitors and research shows that animals fed diets high in trypsin inhibitors over extended periods are prone to develop an enlarged pancreas and pancreatic cancer (Gumbmann, Spangler, Dugan, Rackis, & Liener, (1985).[59] And finally, goitrogens are known to interfere with the production of thyroid hormones by compromising the ability of the thyroid gland to absorb adequate amounts of iodine. Whenever hormone production in any organ in the body is altered, there is always a risk of adverse consequences in other organs in the body that may be regulated by those hormones.

In view of all the health risks associated with soy, one has to wonder why it was considered to be a good choice as food for humans in the first place. It's true that soy has certain nutritional benefits for humans, but it also carries a number of serious health risks. Both USDA and the FDA may have dropped the ball on this one.

Summary

Several decades ago soy was shown to cause pancreatic cancer in animals that were fed soy in long-term feeding trials. Additional research trials have shown that the ingredients known as soy protein isolates that are commonly used in many foods today contain trypsin inhibitors that can cause pancreas enlargement and pancreatic cancer in animal feeding trials.

Soy also contains relatively large amounts of phytic acid. Phytic acid is known to interfere with the absorption of several important minerals, including magnesium. As we determined in chapter 2, magnesium deficiency is associated with a significantly increased risk of PC.

Chapter 8

Fructose and Pancreatic Cancer

Maybe corn syrup, fruit, and fruit juices are not so good for us after all.

Contrary to advertising claims made by certain industry interests, including their paid lobbyists in Washington, D.C., all sugars are not equal. The contention arises around the differences between the ways in which the body processes glucose and fructose.

Sucrose, fructose, and glucose are all simple sugars. Sucrose (aka common table sugar) contains a 50–50 combination of glucose and fructose. By contrast, high fructose corn syrup (HFCS) contains a higher percentage of fructose, and the amount can vary over a wide range depending on individual product specifications. When analyzed for their specific properties, these sugars all provide the same amount of energy per unit of mass. But despite the fact that they contain equal amounts of energy (calories), the ways in which the body utilizes them vary dramatically.

Glucose is the most important sugar (as far as energy production in the body is concerned) and it is also called blood sugar because it's the type primarily used by both the body and the brain as fuel. It can provide all the energy the body and the brain need, although when necessary, both the body and the brain can operate on the conversion of fat into energy.

It's important to note that glucose is the only sugar that triggers an insulin response.

Insulin is produced in response to an increase in the blood glucose level, but an increase in the blood fructose level does not cause an insulin response (Ancira, n.d.).[60] This results in a completely different way of handling fructose metabolization.

Fructose can only be metabolized by the liver, and the process requires the enzyme fructokinase. Insulin allows glucose to pass from the blood into the muscles where it can be immediately burned as fuel. But because fructose does not prompt the release of insulin, fructose will not have the opportunity to be transported to cells where it can be burned as fuel, and because of that important difference, fructose digestion tends to result in the formation of more fat deposits.

Another important difference is the production of leptin.

Leptin is a hormone produced by fat cells and used by the body to regulate energy balance (read that to mean "prevent overeating") by suppressing hunger whenever energy levels are already sufficient. Glucose stimulates the production of leptin, but fructose does not. Obviously the failure to promote the production of leptin creates an increased likelihood of overeating. What does that have to do with pancreatic cancer? According to the American Cancer Society, obesity increases the risk of PC by about 20 % (American Cancer Society, 2016).[61]

Pancreatic cancer uses fructose to rapidly divide and grow new cells.

While it's true that most types of cancer cells tend to thrive on sugar of any type, researchers (Liu et al., 2010) have shown that because of the unique way that fructose is metabolized in the body, pancreatic cancer cells are able to exploit fructose to supercharge their reproductive ability.[62] Liu et al. (2010) made this important observation:

> These findings show that cancer cells can readily metabolize fructose to increase proliferation. They have major significance for cancer patients given dietary refined fructose consumption, and indicate that efforts to reduce refined fructose intake or inhibit fructose-mediated actions may disrupt cancer growth. (p. 6,368)

This implies that avoiding fructose may prevent an existing PC tumor from growing.

This intriguing suggestion by the researchers may have profound significance. Could avoiding fructose in the diet of patients be more effective for treating PC than any of the medical treatments currently available? At the very least, in the light of this discovery, clearly the long-standing claim that all sugars are the same is incorrect.

It seems interesting that PC selects fructose as it's energy source of choice. Could it be that PC makes this selection because of the fact that fructose stimulates neither an insulin response nor the production of leptin? By not triggering an insulin response, fructose is less likely to be burned by the body as a source of energy, thus leaving more for the PC tumor. And by failing to stimulate leptin production, appetite will not be suppressed, so that even more energy will be available if the tumor should need it.

An article in the American Journal of Clinical Nutrition in 2004 revealed that by 1990, the use of high fructose corn syrup in food and drinks had increased by more than 10 times compared with the usage rate 20 years earlier (Bray, Nielsen, & Popkin, 2004).[63] This period of time was associated with what was arguably one of the fastest growing (significant) trends in the human diet to ever occur. Obviously the changes were not as profound as the introduction of wheat, dairy, and grain products at the dawning of the neolithic age, but the diet changes associated with the advent of the neolithic age occurred over many generations (thousands of years) — this one occurred over about 2 or 3 decades (notably, approximately a generation or less). And this change occurred at the same time that the use of soy in human food was being rapidly expanded at similar rates of increase.

Because insulin resistance is involved with magnesium deficiency and diabetes, and both have been shown to be a risk factor for PC, one would think that perhaps diets that are associated with a high glycemic index or a high glycemic load might be associated with a higher risk of PC development. Interestingly, research studies have not been able to find any correlation between glycemic index, total carbohydrates, or glycemic load, and the risk of pancreatic cancer (Jiao et al., 2009).[64] This of course confirms that sugar in general is not a direct PC risk (although it can be an indirect risk by way of contributing to obesity). Fructose is the only sugar that has been shown to significantly increase the risk of developing pancreatic cancer.

Summary

Researchers have discovered that due to the unique way that fructose is metabolized in the body, pancreatic cancer is able to exploit fructose to reproduce and grow rapidly. Despite research showing that fructose enhances the ability of PC to propagate, no evidence has been found that either glycemic index, glycemic load, or total carbohydrates in the diet are associated with an increased PC risk.

Chapter 9

Fat and Pancreatic Cancer

Both dietary fat and higher levels of body fat have been associated with an increased risk of PC.

Does dietary fat significantly affect PC risk? Most published research has been inconclusive. But a relatively large study known as the NI-H-AARP Diet and Health Study claims that fat in the diet does have an effect (Thiébaut et al., 2009).[65] The study found that the strongest correlation was with saturated fat of animal origin, which showed a 43 % increased risk of pancreatic cancer associated with diets that contained the highest amounts of animal fat compared with diets containing the lowest amounts of animal fat.

Interestingly though, when red meat and dairy products were considered separately, the study showed that red meat decreased the risk of PC by 27 %, while dairy products increased the risk by 19 %, both relatively modest amounts. Prior to this report many earlier studies had claimed that eating saturated fats led to various other adverse health risks including obesity, colon cancer and cardiovascular disease.

But sometimes one must take certain research claims with a huge grain of salt because the validity of those claims may depend on who is making the claim, who is paying for the research, and the prevailing medical opinion at the time of the study. The problem lies in the fact that much research data can be analyzed and interpreted in different ways, leading to different conclusions. And researchers sometimes choose to "cherry-pick" data by selecting data that supports a predetermined "plan" for the research project, while rejecting or ignoring data that conflicts with the plan. Various reasons may be listed as justifications for such data selections or omissions, but such methods often significantly alter the conclusions that result from those studies.

For example, an analysis showed that the tallest 1/4 of subjects in a study had a 76 % increased risk of pancreatic cancer compared with the shortest 1/4 of the people in that study (Berrington de González et al., 2006).[66] That's a rather significant risk increase. But that result was based on the fact that the people who were in the shortest category had an unusually low risk of PC. If the researchers ruled out that group (as atypical), that eliminated any differences for the rest. So the way in which the researchers chose to interpret those data made all the difference in the world on how the risk statistics claims appeared in the published report.

But yes, it's true — if you happen to be in the shortest quartile of the general population, then according to published research you have only about half (57 %) of the risk of PC compared with everyone else in the taller categories.

The same study (Berrington de González et al., 2006) also concluded that increasing body mass index has no significant adverse effect on PC risk. And the study also found no evidence that total physical activity significantly decreases the risk of PC. But later studies contradicted the claim that body mass index has no effect on PC risk (as we shall see later in this chapter).

A later study (Aune et al., 2012) concluded that increasing height is associated with a slight increase in the risk of developing pancreatic cancer.[67] But the amount of the increased risk, while large enough to be considered statistically significant in the study, was not large enough to be viewed as a major consideration in comparison with most of the major PC risk factors discussed in this book.

The claim that animal fat in the diet increases the risk of PC is not surprising because at the time of that study (2009), the prevailing consensus of opinion (read that "the popular medical opinion") was still based on the foregone conclusion that eating fat (and especially animal fat) caused obesity, colon cancer, and other health issues such as cardiovascular disease. Like most people, medical researchers and their families like to eat regularly, and because of that habit, rarely can they afford to take a chance on straying very far from officially-endorsed medical policies when writing research articles for prestigious peer-reviewed medical journals.

No one likes to see the publication of medical research that shows that what they have been doing for years in their medical practice is just plain wrong. When a research article is submitted for publication, if any of the medical authorities doing the peer reviews happen to be less than totally objective, and they choose to disallow a researcher's articles repeatedly, that researcher may soon find her or himself unable to secure funding for future research, effectively ending their chances of advancing in their research career (to say nothing of jeopardizing their chances of putting food on the table by means of gainful employment as a researcher).

Because of that risk, most research reports are not likely to stray very far from conventional thinking unless the researchers are willing to risk being secretly "blacklisted". Of course few people in the industry care to talk about such problems, but the overall effects on research are considerable, and they can have long-term effects on the direction of research. And obviously such an environment tends to serve as a deterrent for progress when the research discoveries contradict current medical thinking.

Nonetheless, in very recent years, studies have been published that examined that same original research data, and the newer studies dispute many of the conclusions claimed by those earlier research articles. For example, a study of dairy fat consumption published in 2016 was based on data retrieved from 9 databases in 15 different countries, involving 636,151 different patients, spanning a period of 6.5 million person-years of follow-up. This newer study resulted in a totally different conclusion that contradicts the claims stated in earlier studies. Pimpin, Wu, Haskelberg, Del Gobbo, and Mozaffarian (2016) concluded that the consumption of butter had only a neutral to a small (relatively insignificant) effect on mortality, cardiovascular disease, and diabetes.[68] They found no justification for dietary guidelines (either pro or con) regarding the consumption of butter.

Replacing animal fat in the diet with plant-based fat does not reduce mortality risks.

Other recent research has shown that replacing animal fat in the diet with plant-based polyunsaturated fatty acids such as linoleic acid tends to lower the blood cholesterol level but it does not reduce the risk of death from coronary heart disease, nor does it reduce all-cause mortality risk (Ramsden et al., 2016).[69]

So clearly, conventional thinking is beginning to shift in recent years because these studies are being successfully published in prestigious medical journals. But does this prove that animal fat is not associated with an increased risk of PC, implying that the study published by Berrington de González et al. (2006) is invalid? Certainly not. But it does raise some questions about the ways in which the data may have been selected and analyzed in the study.

For example, did the researchers omit any data that disagreed with their conclusions? Or could the published results have been influenced by the mainstream medical community's bias against animal fat in the diet that prevailed at the time? Because the study was specifically targeted at pancreatic cancer, and it was a huge study, we certainly cannot simply write it off as meaningless unless more recent research studies offer more compelling evidence to the contrary, specifically related to the risk of developing PC.

Does body weight or obesity have an effect on PC risk?

According to a study published by Stolzenberg-Solomon, Schairer, Moore, Hollenbeck, and Silverman (2013), being overweight does increase the risk of developing pancreatic cancer.[70] The researchers found that a condition of overweight or obesity was associated with an increased risk of PC that ranged from 15 to 53 %. And not surprisingly, the study results showed that the higher risk levels were associated with being overweight for longer periods of time.

In general, for every 10 years associated with a body mass index (BMI) greater than 25, there was a 6 % increase in the risk of PC. For those who also had diabetes, every 10 years associated with a body mass index greater than 25 increased the risk of PC by 18 %.

Another study focused on body mass index alone showed similar results.

Jiao et al. (2010) showed that compared with a normal BMI in the range from 18.5–25, BMI ratings in the range from 25–30 were associated with a 13 % increased risk of PC.[71] Similarly, BMI ratings in the range from 30–35 were associated with a 19 % increased risk of PC. Obviously these are rather modest increases in risk levels. An earlier study (Stolzenberg-Solomon et al., 2008) based on a cohort of 302, 060 subjects, concluded that BMI ratings of 35 or above were associated with a 45 % increased PC risk.[72] This study also found no association between PC and physical activity levels.

Summary

Studies show that both dietary fat (especially animal fat) and excess body fat are associated with an increased risk of PC. However, more recently published studies have shown that the conclusions reported in many earlier studies were biased, and unfairly targeted animal fat as the cause of obesity, colon cancer, and cardiovascular disease when in fact the data do not support such claims. This raises a possible question about the accuracy of reports (especially older published articles) that claim a large increase in PC risk associated with the consumption of animal fat.

It's possible that the claims may be exaggerated. Even so, in the absence of convincing evidence that specifically discredits the claims, it may be prudent to assume that they might be correct until proven otherwise. After all, pancreatic cancer is a very unforgiving disease.

To add to the confusion, later studies contradicted the earlier claims that body mass index has no significant effect on PC risk. One of the studies even showed increasing risk ratings for increasing BMI levels.

Chapter 10

Odds and Ends and Pancreatic Cancer

Various types of issues have been studied in an attempt to track down critical links to PC.

Family history has long been known to be a risk factor for pancreatic cancer. Jacobs et al. (2010) conducted an extensive analysis to determine that when a parent, sibling, or child had been previously diagnosed with PC, that increased a person's risk of PC by 76 %.[73] Other factors that appear to affect the risk of PC include pancreatitis (inflammation of the pancreas), which has been shown to increase the risk of PC by 368 %, and smoking (Maisonneuve et al., 2010).[74] Heavy smokers who have a family history of pancreatitis have been shown by the same study (Maisonneuve et al., 2010) to have 15.4 times the risk of PC when compared with control cases in the study. Similar to the indications that in some cases Type 2 diabetes may be a symptom of pancreatic cancer, (as we discussed back in chapter 3) Maisonneuve et al. (2010) suggested that the possibility exists that pancreatitis may in some cases be an early indicator of PC.

It's been said that every cloud has a silver lining. That silver lining may apply to allergies, because the study by Maisonneuve et al. (2010) also revealed that people in the study who had a history of allergies, had a reduced risk of PC that was 36 % less than the risk for people who did not have a history of allergies.

A large study showed that an increased risk of PC is less likely with type O blood than with any other type (Amundadottir et al., 2009).[75] The study by Amundadottir et al. (2009) suggested that blood types other than type O carried a 20 % increased PC risk. But another large study carried the research even farther and concluded that compared with type O, blood type A was associated with a 38 % increased risk of PC, type AB was associated with a 47 % increased risk, and type B was linked with a 53 % increased risk (Wolpin et al., 2010).[76]

In a study of 470,681 subjects, Jiao et al. (2009) found that alcohol consumption increases PC risk.[77] Compared with light drinkers (less than 1 drink per day average), those who had 3 or more drinks per day had a 45 % increased risk of PC. Heavy liquor users in the study had a 62 % increased risk. But because it's well-established that alcohol consumption depletes magnesium (Flink, 1986), this association between higher alcohol consumption rates and higher PC risk may be due (at least in part) to magnesium deficiency.

As we learned in chapters 2 and 3, insulin resistance appears to be associated with the development of PC. And some authorities have often speculated that sugar use may play a role in PC risk. But a study of 487,922 subjects by Bao et al. (2008). could not find any significant evidence of a connection between sugar intake and pancreatic cancer risk.[78]

A huge study by Guertin et al. (2015) involving 4,155,156 subject years showed no significant association between total coffee intake and PC.[79] And this held true for both caffeinated and decaffeinated coffee.

Summary

A family history of PC increases the risk of PC development, and some blood types carry an increased risk of PC. While increasing alcohol intake has an adverse effect on PC risk, coffee consumption does not appear to affect PC risk, and neither does sugar intake (although some of the effects of sugar intake such as obesity can increase PC risk). And a history of allergies actually lowers the risk of PC when compared with people who do not have a history of allergies.

Chapter 11

Looking at a Couple of Case Studies

Certain case studies provide some interesting insight into the realities of pancreatic cancer.

No process in this world can be assumed to be 100 % effective, but dietary changes are not only very effective for preventing cancer, but also many other health issues. And similarly, proper diet changes can also be very effective for treating existing disease.

Let's consider a real world case with which most people are at least somewhat familiar. Arguably the most popular celebrity to become a victim of PC in recent times (as of the date of publication of this book) is Steve Jobs. Jobs had an uncommon form of PC known as a neuroendocrine tumor. Approximately 5 % of PC cases involve this type which grows and spreads much more slowly than the more common form known as pancreatic adenocarcinoma (Gardner, n.d.).[80] Neuroendocrine tumors develop in a certain type of cells in the pancreas known as islet cells. The purpose of these cells is to produce hormones to regulate certain body functions.

The more common pancreatic adenocarcinomas develop in the ductal cells that line the drainage tubes of the pancreas, and these tumors tend to be much more aggressive than the neuroendocrine type. Pancreatic adenocarcinomas are the type that are typically referred to as simply "pancreatic cancer". Because Jobs had the type that grows much more slowly (a neuroendocrine tumor), he survived for 8 years after it was diagnosed in 2003.

But apparently he had the cancer for many years before it was diagnosed.

The fact that it was a slow-growing tumor allowed for some interesting observations. His surgery in 2004 revealed that the cancer had already spread to his liver.

Dr. John McDougall used the diameter of the liver tumor to work backwards to calculate the growth rate for the cancer and used that to extrapolate that the cancer had probably spread to the liver approximately 7 years earlier (McDougall, 2011, November).[81] So that suggests that Jobs lived at least 15 years with pancreatic cancer, after it had spread to his liver. Obviously that implies that the pancreatic cancer would have had to originate at least several years prior to that because cancers typically do not metastasize until after they have developed for at least several years.

Other information from the past, such as a report indicating that in 1987 his hands had a yellow appearance, add support to the probability that the tumor had existed for many years, because that issue occurred approximately 24 years before his death. Jaundice is a well-known side effect of PC in some cases. Using this and other information, Dr. McDougall estimated that the pancreatic cancer may have originated when Jobs was in his early to mid-twenties, roughly 30 years before he died.

This suggests that the vegan and sometimes fruitarian diet that Jobs followed might have slowed down the growth of the tumor. But the problem is that the evidence suggests that this diet also helped to create a virtually ideal environment for the development of PC.

There's a reason for everything that happens.

Now that you have finished reading in this book about most of the known dietary issues that increase the risk of pancreatic cancer, you can clearly understand why Jobs had a high risk of developing pancreatic cancer, and why the tumor apparently began when he was at a relatively young age.

The first clue goes back to his youth when he was reportedly plagued by body odor (Mertz, 2014).[82] Most people have just assumed that this problem was due to not bathing often enough. And it's true that after he adopted a fruit and vegetable diet he decided that his diet made him immune to body odor so he stopped bathing regularly.

But it appears that the body odor problem was present long before he changed his bathing habits.

His strong body odor is the reason why he began eating a vegan diet. He thought that the diet would eliminate the problem. He eventually decided that his diet was so effective at controlling body odor that he could afford to skip bathing. At any rate, it certainly isn't clear that failure to bathe often enough was the initial cause of the odor when he was younger. So please allow me to offer my personal viewpoint (based on my own experiences), which completely differs from the popular assumption that his body odor was always (and solely) due to poor hygiene.

Jobs' early body odor issues were almost certainly caused by a magnesium deficiency.

I have personally experienced not only a chronic magnesium deficiency, but also an acute (severe) magnesium deficiency brought on when a series of 3 back-to-back antibiotic treatments for dental work depleted what was left of my meager reserves of magnesium, and caused a serious magnesium deficiency. In addition to all of the debilitating symptoms that can sometimes occur when the autonomic nervous system is unable to perform normally, so that it becomes incapable of properly regulating vital body functions, I would wake up in the wee hours of the morning, sweating profusely (even though the room was very cool), and the disgusting odor of the fluids flowing out of my pores seemed toxic enough to knock a buzzard off a garbage truck at least half a mile away. The timing was almost surely determined by the likelihood that this was when my body would run out of magnesium because the amount of magnesium in the last meal had been used up by then. Like Steve Jobs, I found that odor to be extremely offensive and intolerable.

I had never smelled anything like it before (nor since), but now I would recognize it immediately if exposed to it again. Because my doctors were unable to make the connection between all my symptoms and the cause, this went on for weeks before I finally figured it out myself and resolved it by increasing my magnesium intake.

Magnesium deficiency is a widespread problem that physicians simply do not recognize (because they're not trained to recognize it and they have no experience in recognizing it). The Emergency Room doctors even missed mine when I went there after my symptoms eventually became so severe that I couldn't force myself to eat breakfast one morning. When I went to the ER, my heart rate was way too high and my blood pressure was up in the "stroke risk" range. My blood sugar was high (because magnesium deficiency causes insulin resistance), and a serum

68

magnesium test result was below range, and it was even flagged by the lab. In addition, my estimated glomerular filtration rate (EGFR) test result was flagged as significantly below normal (because magnesium deficiency compromises kidney function).

And yet the doctors there assured me that my test results were "fine" and there was nothing apparently wrong with me, and they sent me back home. Fortunately I checked my test results online a couple of days later and I recognized what the flagged test results meant. But those test results apparently meant nothing to the ER doctors because they are not trained to look for, nor to recognize magnesium deficiency symptoms and lab test markers.

So my point is that if magnesium deficiency was initially the cause of Jobs' body odor problems when he was young, or even part of the cause in later years, then his doctors would almost certainly never have caught the connection.

As pointed out in chapter 2 (page 19), research shows that genetics can compromise the ability of some individuals to absorb magnesium, so he could have been born with a predisposition for magnesium deficiency. The odds of that deficiency ever being diagnosed by his doctors were virtually nil.

Another clue was his apparent problems with kidney stones. I can verify by personal experience that a magnesium deficiency causes significant kidney problems. It can cause frequent urination, and urgent urination. The only kidney stones I ever had in my life showed up approximately 6 months before my increasing magnesium deficiency symptoms became severe enough to cause me to make that visit to the ER described a couple of pages earlier. And as I noted in my description of that ER visit, magnesium deficiency can interfere with kidney function resulting in below range EGFR lab test results.

Kidney problems were presumably the reason why Jobs had the scan in 2003 that revealed the spot on his pancreas that lead to his PC diagnosis. But apparently he had been dealing with kidney issues for years. So there are plenty of reasons to suspect that he may have been magnesium deficient for many years, probably going all the way back to his childhood.

And then there was his diet.

Jobs' diet was unusual, to say the least (Daniel, 2011, December 27, Dahl, 2011, November 2).[83,84] As any dietitian will quickly point out, Jobs' high-carb diet deprived his body of protein and fat. It's possible to not only survive, but be quite healthy with absolutely no carbs in the diet, but protein and fat are both essential to good health, especially the health of vital organs. Without adequate protein he was almost surely short of some of the essential amino acids.

And if at least 15 % of one's calories does not come from fat, not only is there a huge risk of a deficiency of essential fatty acids, but deficiencies of the fat-soluble vitamins (A, D, E, and K) are also likely to develop (Bruso, 2015, May 1).[85] That leads to weakened organs, and most importantly, a weakened immune system.

And you have probably already spotted the other major problem with Jobs' diet — fruit (and fruit juice) and vegetables are loaded with fructose. McDougall (2011, November), credited Jobs' diet with extending his life (which may or may not be true).

Steve Jobs getting cancer was an unfortunate accident—like being struck by lightning or hit by a car. The carcinogen(s) entered his body and due to genetics, "bad luck," or other unknown and uncontrollable factors his body was susceptible. The cause of his cancer was not due to his vegan diet. In fact, his healthy diet likely slowed the growth of his tumor, delayed the time of diagnosis, and prolonged his useful life.

But in that 2011 article McDougall also absolved the diet of any guilt in Job's death and that claim clearly flies in the face of what we now know about the risks associated with the development of pancreatic cancer. Was he correct? You be the judge.

While it's probably true that no one will ever prove that the diet was singularly responsible for the development of the cancer that eventually took Steve Jobs' life, there's no question that the diet helped to create an arguably ideal environment for the development of pancreatic cancer. Between the apparent magnesium deficiency, the likely amino acid deficiencies, the fatty acids and fat-soluble vitamin deficiencies (especially the vitamin D deficiency), together with the high-fructose component of his diet, Jobs' body was exceptionally vulnerable to PC. In retrospect, if someone set out to develop an optimal diet that maximized the opportunity for the development and growth of pancreatic cancer, they would arguably be hard put to find a better way to go about it than to follow Job's unusual diet.

The main point here is that without such a severely-weakened immune system (as a result of the diet), a carcinogen entering the body might have been a moot point, because the immune system would have probably destroyed any malignant cells before they could become established. But a compromised immune system cannot perform well, and therein lies the problem. A compromised immune system is often unable to adequately protect the body from pathogens that would have normally been routinely destroyed.

71

Dr. Josh Axe, a naturopathic practitioner, has suggested that Jobs might have lived much longer if he had not had a liver transplant (2 years prior to his death). The organ transplant required that Jobs take an immune system suppressant for the rest of his life in order to prevent his immune system from rejecting the transplanted liver (Axe, 2011).[86]

The point is that without a functioning immune system, Jobs no longer had a way to fight cancer. And of course that observation makes sense. Axe also points out that most people choose to stick with conventional (allopathic) medical treatments such as radiation, chemotherapy, and drugs to treat their PC, and they tend to survive for only a few months after their diagnosis.

The logic of Dr. Axe's observations cannot be denied. Without a fully-functional immune system, the human body is a sitting duck target for virtually any pathogen that comes along. The powerful immune system suppressants used after organ transplants virtually turn off the immune system.

And while chemotherapy is generally considered to be somewhat less of a threat because it is typically thought to only suppresses the immune system during the treatment period (and for a short time afterward), the risk is significantly greater than is generally realized. Recent research shows that recovery of the immune system from chemotherapy treatment can take up to 9 months (Verma et al., 2016, January 26).[87] Radiation treatment usually carries less of a threat to the immune system, but it can still compromise some aspects of the immune system.

Dr. Ralph Steinman was a well-known Canadian immunologist.

By a cruel twist of irony, he died of pancreatic cancer in the fall of 2011 just 3 days before the Nobel committee made a phone call to inform him that he had won the Nobel Prize for his work in immunology (Altman & Wade, 2011, October 3).[88] But he had the aggressive form of PC known as adenocarcinoma. While it's not unusual for neuroendocrine cancer patients to live for years or even decades with the disease, that's not the case for pancreatic adenocarcinoma patients. With this aggressive form of cancer, life expectancy after diagnosis is typically measured in months.

In sharp contrast with Jobs' (unintentional) immune system-crippling diet, and his forced use of an immune system suppressing drug (because of the liver transplant), Dr. Steinman's approach was to do everything possible to boost the effectiveness of his immune system so that it could fight the tumor. By doing so, he was able to survive for a very impressive total of 4 years, mostly because of the use of vaccines based on his own research, and the use of other experimental medical treatments (Gravitz, 2011, October 11, Engber, 2012, December 21, Cancer Research Institute, n.d.).[89,90,91]

An important point to remember from this is that both of these patients survived for an unusually long time (for their respective forms of PC), apparently because they used unconventional treatment techniques. But eventually pancreatic cancer took their lives anyway, despite desperate efforts to stop it.

We have no information on Dr. Steinman's nutritional status prior to his development of PC, but the evidence strongly suggests that Steve Jobs may have been magnesium deficient during his adolescent years and possibly earlier than that. We have no way of knowing for sure. He might have been born with genetics that compromised his ability to absorb magnesium. And his vegan/ fruitarian (fat-deficient) diet almost surely resulted in a deficiency of at least some of the fat-soluble vitamins (such as vitamins A, D, E, and K), over the long term. A vitamin D deficiency in particular is known to severely weaken the immune sys-

73

tem's ability to defend the body from pathogenic invaders. Whatever the case, it appears that prevention is still by far the most effective way available for most people to prevent becoming another statistic of pancreatic cancer.

Summary
Conventional cancer treatments, including treatments for pancreatic cancer, typically involve methods that tend to suppress the immune system, which is generally counterproductive for fighting disease. Suppressing a patient's immune system can allow organisms that would ordinarily not pose a serious threat, (because the immune system could easily destroy them) to become life-threatening under certain circumstances.

But alternative cancer treatments, which typically involve methods that include dietary changes, fasting, colon cleansing and related practices, also tend to contain possibly fatal flaws. They often include a high-fructose diet and/or they involve methods that weaken the immune system by further depleting already deficient levels of magnesium and vitamin D.

Chapter 12

Recent Research Discoveries

While research shows promise in some areas, progress against PC remains slow.

Conventional wisdom adheres to the opinion that pancreatic cancer is so lethal because it is very aggressive. But according to Dr. Bert Vogelstein of the Howard Hughes Medical Institute, who participated in a study that was published in 2010, that is not actually the case (Howard Hughes Medical Institute, 2010, October 27, Yachida et al., 2010).[92,93] Their research showed that many pancreatic cancer tumors actually grow very slowly, typically developing over a period of approximately 20 years before they pose a lethal threat. The reason why they are so lethal is simply because they are typically diagnosed only after they have been growing so long that they have metastasized to other organs. And similar to most other types of cancer, it is the tumors that have spread to other organs that are the primary cause of death with PC.

This allows plenty of time for a diagnosis while the disease is still at a stage that could be easily treated. The problem is that so far at least, medical science has been unable to figure out a way to diagnose PC before it causes symptoms, and typically, symptoms do not develop until after the cancer has spread to other organs. By then, the window of opportunity for treatment success may no longer be available.

8 Ways to Prevent Pancreatic Cancer

Natural treatments are appealing to many patients because they tend to eliminate the side effect risks so common with conventional cancer treatments. Some research has been done using curcumin to treat pancreatic cancer cells in laboratory settings. And a relatively small study indicated that curcumin was about as effective as chemotherapy for treating PC patients (Ranjan, Mukerjee, Helson, Gupta, & Vishwanatha, 2013, Dhillon et al., 2008, Kanai, 2014).[94,95,96]

Unfortunately, chemotherapy is not very effective against PC, but at least a curcumin treatment avoids the side effect risks of chemotherapy, so it holds some promise for possible future treatment options. One of the biggest problems with many conventional cancer treatments is that they tend to destroy the ability of the immune system to perform normally, thus leaving the body defenseless against infection and disease.

Gains using conventional treatments continue to be small. For example, researchers have determined that by using a combination of drugs (gemcitabine plus capecitabine), a 15 % improvement in 5-year survival rates can be gained, compared with using gemcitabine alone (Mulcahy, 2016, June 4).[97]

Some pancreatic cancer-related research focuses on reducing the incidence of Type 2 diabetes. This is of interest because Type 2 diabetes is so closely linked with an increased risk of PC. Satija et al. (2016) for example showed that a plant-based diet with reduced intake of animal-based food resulted in a significant reduction in the risk of developing Type 2 diabetes.[98]

However, while that article (Satija et al., 2016) specifically mentions the benefits of magnesium in glucose metabolism, and points out that a plant-based diet is likely to contain increased amounts of magnesium, it appears that no effort was made to screen out or identify magnesium-deficient subjects in the study. Nor was there any effort made to rate the magnesium deficiency or sufficiency of the subjects in any way. Multi-vitamin use was noted, but virtually all multivitamins contain magnesium oxide as their primary source of magnesium, and it's well established that magnesium oxide is the least likely form of magnesium to be absorbed out of all the magnesium supplementation options available.

So tracking multivitamins but not tracking magnesium supplements used in the study provided data of limited value.

Because magnesium deficiency is a strong independent risk factor for the development of insulin resistance and Type 2 diabetes, the research data may have been confounded by the failure of the researchers to consider magnesium deficiency as a confounding factor.

This is an important point because it's possible that because the researchers failed to properly correlate data from magnesium-deficient subjects in the study, the data may be seriously skewed. It's possible that the increased level of magnesium in plant-based diets may have been the primary reason why the study showed that plant-based diets reduced the number of cases of Type 2 diabetes. And if that is the case, then magnesium supplementation would be more important for preventing Type 2 diabetes than utilizing plant-based diets. In other words, the fact that the researchers ignored the influence of magnesium deficiency on the data suggests that they may have simply been trying to promote a plant-based diet over an animal-based diet.

For example, Rumawas et al. (2006) concluded that in their study, the mechanism by which increased magnesium intake reduced the risk of developing Type 2 diabetes appeared to be associated with improving insulin sensitivity.[99] This claim was supported by additional research publications. As discussed on page 26, back in chapter 3, Hruby et al. (2014) showed that people in their study who had the highest magnesium intake had only about half the risk (53 %) of metabolic impairment or diabetes development compared with those who had the lowest magnesium intake. By comparison, the study by Satija et al. (2016) showed benefits in a numerically similar range for plant-based diets compared with animal-based diets. That suggests that the benefits shown by Satija et al. (2016) might possibly have been almost entirely due to increased magnesium intake in the diets of subjects in the study who followed plant-based diets. That possibility raises some serious questions about the validity of not only the data used in the plant-based diet versus animal-based diet study, but also the conclusions reached in that study.

But while researchers, USDA, and various other health authorities continue to promote diets that contain more fruit and vegetables, the trend among American consumers continues in the opposite direction. Perhaps this is associated with the trend toward decreased use of sugar and especially HFCS in processed foods. Fruit juice consumption and fruit and vegetable consumption is declining, according to USDA data (Lin, & Morrison, 2016, July 5).[100] Does this imply that fructose consumption may be declining as well? Maybe this trend is not so bad after all. Perhaps consumers know what is best for them and they don't need government "experts" wasting taxpayer money to tell them what to eat.

Dr. Harald zur Hausen was jointly awarded the Nobel Prize in physiology or medicine in 2008.

He received the award for his work in discovering that the human papillomaviruses HPV 16 and HPV 18 are responsible for cervical cancer. The contributions of his research team eventually led to the development of the vaccine that became available in 2006. But he proposed the original theory back in 1976. It took 7 years for his team of researchers to determine that HPV 16 and HPV 18 were the strains that can lead to cervical cancer. So it took 30 years to get from a theory to a vaccine available for use by the public.

Dr. Hausen has another very interesting theory that he and his team are now investigating. Whether or not this theory might apply to pancreatic cancer remains to be seen, but there appears to be a good chance that it might, because if his theory can be proven, that would raise the percentage of cancer cases that can be caused by an infectious agent to 35 %, a sizable increase from the current 20 % level. Dr. Hausen has proposed that colon cancer is caused by a virus common in beef cattle (Wang, 2015, February 2).[101]

And he cites some very good arguments to support his theory. But as was the case with his previous award-winning work, it will surely take many years before the theory can be either proven or ruled out. If the theory turns out to be correct however, that would surely prompt an increased level of research to search for a viral or bacterial infectious link for pancreatic cancer.

Some research articles have suggested a connection between H. pylori infections and the development of PC, but research results so far have been inconclusive. It has also been suggested that H. pylori may be implicated in the development of autoimmune pancreatitis (Bulajic, Panic, & Löhr, 2014).[102] There is a very good chance that this observation may someday prove to be an important finding. We've already noted back in chapter 10, on page 61, that pancreatitis can more than quadruple the risk of pancreatic cancer.

But until the medical community discovers or develops methods for diagnosing pancreatic cancer long before it spreads to other organs, prevention will continue to offer the best hope for avoiding becoming a statistic of the disease. And the best time to begin making the lifestyle changes that you feel can be helpful for protecting you from pancreatic cancer without seriously disrupting your chosen lifestyle, is right now, today.

Summary

While researchers continue to study associations between PC and various possible causative agents, precious little progress is being made where it really counts, namely in finding ways to allow diagnosis of the disease while it is still in a treatable stage (before it has metastasized). There is always hope that some unforeseen breakthrough may occur, but as long as the prevailing attitude regarding approved treatment methods continues to focus on procedures that tend to weaken the immune system, it's difficult to visualize any dramatic breakthroughs in mainstream medical treatment methods for PC, or any other type of cancer. Additional small steps in treatment improvements will surely be made, but mainstream medicine desperately needs to step back and reassess the way in which not only pancreatic cancer, but cancer in general is viewed.

When current treatment methods are ineffective, or only marginally effective, it's time to do some thinking outside the box. Continuing to use the same ineffective approach to a problem can only result in a continuation of relatively poor results.

About the Author

Wayne Persky BSME

Wayne Persky was born, grew up, and currently lives in Central Texas. He is a graduate of the University of Texas at Austin, College of Engineering, with postgraduate studies in mechanical engineering, mathematics, and computer science. He has teaching experience in engineering, and business experience in farming and agribusiness.

After the onset of severe digestive system and general health problems in the late 1990s, he went through extensive clinical testing, but the GI specialist failed to take biopsies during a colonoscopy exam, and even failed to test for celiac disease. Afterward, not surprisingly, he was told by his gastroenterologist that there was nothing wrong with him.

Unable to find a medical solution, he was forced to use his research skills to discover innovative ways to resolve his health issues. After extensive study, he identified the likely source of the problem as food sensitivities.

It took a year and a half of avoiding all traces of gluten, plus trial and error experimentation with other foods, and careful record-keeping, to track down all of the food issues. But once he eliminated all of them from his diet, he got his life back. He currently administrates an online microscopic colitis discussion and support forum, while continuing to live on a farm in Central Texas. In 2015 he founded the Microscopic Colitis Foundation and he continues to serve as president and as a contributing author to the Newsletter.

Contact Details:

Wayne Persky can be contacted at:
Persky Farms
19242 Darrs Creek Rd
Bartlett, TX 76511
USA

Tel: 1(254)718-1125
Tel: 1(254)527-3682

Email: wayne@perskyfarms.com

For information and support regarding microscopic colitis, visit:

http://www.microscopiccolitisfoundation.org/

To participate in the Discussion and Support Forum go to:

http://www.perskyfarms.com/phpBB2/index.php

My author website can be found at http://www.waynepersky.com/

Alphabetical Index

Alphabetical Index

8 Ways to Prevent Pancreatic Cancer

1 Gudjonsson, B. (1987). Cancer of the pancreas. 50 years of surgery. *Cancer, 60*(9), 2284-303. Retrieved from http://www.ncbi.nlm.nih.gov/pubmed/3326653

2 The Sol Goldman Pancreatic Cancer Research Center. (2015). Johns Hopkins University [Web log message]. Retrieved from http://pathology.jhu.edu/pc/basicintro.php?area=ba

3 Pancreatic cancer to become second-leading cause of cancer death by 2020. (2012, November 9). Imaging Technology News [Web log message]. Retrieved from http://www.itnonline.com/content/pancreatic-cancer-become-second-leading-cause-cancer-death-2020

4 Dall'igna, P., Cecchetto, G., Bisogno, G., Conte, M., Chiesa, P. L., D'Angelo, P. . . . TREP Group. (2010). Pancreatic tumors in children and adolescents: the Italian TREP project experience. *Pediatric Blood & Cancer, 54*(5), 675-680. Retrieved from http://www.ncbi.nlm.nih.gov/pubmed/19998473

5 Dibaba, D., Xun, P., Yokota, K., White, E., & He, K. (2015). Magnesium intake and incidence of pancreatic cancer: The VITamins and Lifestyle study. *British Journal of Cancer, 113*(11), 1612–1621. Retrieved from http://www.ncbi.nlm.nih.gov/pubmed/26554653

6 Magnesium Fact Sheet for Health Professionals. (2016, February 11). National Institutes of Health Office of Dietary Supplements [Web log message]. Retrieved from https://ods.od.nih.gov/factsheets/Magnesium-HealthProfessional/

7 Mauskop, A., & Varughese, J. (2012). Why all migraine patients should be treated with magnesium. *Journal of Neural Transmission (Vienna), 119*(5), 575-579. Retrieved from http://www.ncbi.nlm.nih.gov/pubmed/22426836

8 Persky, W. (2013). Vitamin D and Autoimmune Disease. Bartlett, TX: Persky Farms.

9 Flink, E. B. (1986). Magnesium deficiency in alcoholism. Alcoholism: Clinical and Experimental Research, 10(6), 590-594. Retrieved from www.ncbi.nlm.nih.gov/pubmed/3544909

10 FDA Drug Safety Communication: (2011, March 2). Low magnesium levels can be associated with long-term use of proton pump inhibitor drugs (PPIs). U.S. Food and Drug Administration [Web log message]. Retrieved from http://www.fda.gov/Drugs/DrugSafety/ucm245011.htm

11 Magnesium. (n.d.). University of Maryland Medical Center, [Web log message]. Retrieved from http://umm.edu/health/medical/altmed/supplement/magnesium

12 Sircus, M. (2009, December 8). Magnesium thirst magnesium hunger [Web log message]. Retrieved from http://drsircus.com/medicine/magnesium/magnesium-deficien-cy-symptoms-diagnosis

13 Schachter, M. B. (1996). The importance of magnesium to human nutrition [Web log message]. Retrieved from http://www.mbschachter.-com/importance_of_magnesium_to_human.htm

14 Gilliland, F. D., Berhane K. T., Li, Y. F., Kim, D. H., & Margolis, H. G. (2002). Dietary magnesium, potassium, sodium, and children's lung function. *American Journal of Epidemiology, 155*(2), 125-31. Retrieved from http://www.ncbi.nlm.nih.gov/pubmed/11790675

15 Nuytten, D., Van Hees, J., Meulemans, A., & Carton, H. (1991). Magnesium deficiency as a cause of acute intractable seizures. *Journal of Neurology, 238*(5), 262-264. Retrieved from http://www.ncbi.nlm.nih.-

gov/pubmed/1919610

16 Yuen, A.W., & Sander, J. W. (2012). Can magnesium supplementation reduce seizures in people with epilepsy? A hypothesis. *Epilepsy Research, 100*(1-2), 152-156. Retrieved from http://www.ncbi.nlm.nih.gov/pubmed/22406257

17 Galland, L. (1991–1992). Magnesium, stress and neuropsychiatric disorders. *Magnesium and Trace Elements 10*(2-4), 287-301. Retrieved from http://www.ncbi.nlm.nih.gov/pubmed/1844561

18 King, D. E., Mainous III, A. G., Geesey, M. E., Egan, B. M., & Rehman, S. (2006). Magnesium supplement intake and C-reactive protein levels in adults. *Nutrition Research 26*(5), 193–196. Retrieved from http://www.nrjournal.com/article/S0271-5317%2806%2900092-3/abstract?cc=y

19 Eby, G. A., & Eby, K. L. (2006). Rapid recovery from major depression using magnesium treatment. *Medical Hypotheses, 67*(2), 362–370. Retrieved from http://www.ncbi.nlm.nih.gov/pubmed/16542786

20 Batabyal, P., Vander Hoorn, S., Christophi, C., & Nikfarjam, M. (2014). *Association of Diabetes Mellitus and Pancreatic Adenocarcinoma: A Meta-Analysis of 88 Studies. Annals of Surgical Oncology, Volume 21*(7). Retrieved from http://www.annsurgoncol.org/journals/abstract.html?v=21&j=10434&i=7&a=3625_10.1245_s10434-014-3625-6&doi=

21 Wang, F., Herrington, M., Larsson, J., & Permert, J. (2003). The relationship between diabetes and pancreatic cancer. *Molecular Cancer, 2*(4). Retrieved from http://www.ncbi.nlm.nih.gov/pmc/articles/PMC149418/

22 Gullo, L., Pezzilli, R., Morselli-Labate, A. M., & the Italian Pancreatic Cancer Study Group. (1994). Diabetes and the Risk of Pancreatic Can-

cer. *The New England Journal of Medicine, 331,* 81-84. Retrieved from
http://www.nejm.org/doi/full/10.1056/NEJM199407143310203

23 Schwarts, S. S., Zeidler, A., Moossa, A. R., Kuku, S. F., & Rubenstein,
A. H. (1978). A prospective study of glucose tolerance, insulin, C-pep-
tide, and glucagon responses in patients with pancreatic carcinoma.
The American Journal of Digestive Diseases, 23(12):1107-14. Retrieved
from http://www.ncbi.nlm.nih.gov/pubmed/367155s

24 Permert, J., Adrian, T. E., Jacobsson, P., Jorfelt, L., Fruin, A. B., & Larsson, J. (1993). Is profound peripheral insulin resistance in patients
with pancreatic cancer caused by a tumor-associated factor? *American
Journal of Surgery, 165*(1), 61-6. Retrieved from
http://www.ncbi.nlm.nih.gov/pubmed/8380314

25 Everhart, J., & Wright, D. (1995). Diabetes mellitus as a risk factor for
pancreatic cancer. A meta-analysis. *The Journal of the American Medical
Association, 273*(20), 1605-1609. Retrieved from
http://www.ncbi.nlm.nih.gov/pubmed/7745774

26 Takaya, J., Higashino, H., & Kobayashi, Y. (2004). Intracellular magnesium and insulin resistance. *Magnesium Research, 17*(2), 126-136. Retrieved from http://www.ncbi.nlm.nih.gov/pubmed/15319146

27 Sircus, M. (2009, December 8). The Insulin Magnesium Story [Web
log message]. Retrieved from http://drsircus.com/medicine/magne-
sium/the-insulin-magnesium-story-2

28 Hruby, A., Meigs, J. B., O'Donnell, C. J., Jacques, P. F., & McKeown,
N. M. (2014). Higher Magnesium Intake Reduces Risk of Impaired
Glucose and Insulin Metabolism and Progression From Prediabetes
to Diabetes in Middle-Aged Americans. Diabetes Care, 37(2), 419-427.
Retrieved from http://care.diabetesjournals.org/content/37/2/419

29 Langley, W. F., & Mann, D. (1991). Central nervous system magnesium deficiency. *Archives of Internal Medicine, 151*(3), 593-596. Retrieved from http://www.ncbi.nlm.nih.gov/pubmed/2001142

30 Hjalgrim, H., Frisch, M., Ekbom, A., Kyvik, K. O., Melbye, M., & Green, A. (1997). Cancer and diabetes--a follow-up study of two population-based cohorts of diabetic patients. *Journal of Internal Medicine, 241*(6), 471–475. Retrieved from http://www.ncbi.nlm.nih.gov/pubmed/10497622

31 Zong, G., Eisenberg, D. M., Hu, F. B., & Sun, Q. (2016). Consumption of meals prepared at home and risk of type 2 diabetes: An analysis of two prospective cohort studies. PLOS Medicine. Retrieved from http://dx.doi.org/10.1371/journal.pmed.1002052

32 Editorial Staff. (2016, July 5). Enjoying meals prepared at home: Short-cut to avoiding diabetes? ScienceDaily [Web log message] Retrieved from https://www.sciencedaily.com/releases/2016/07/160705144054.htm

33 Ramsden, C. E., Zamora, D., Majchrzak-Hong, S., Faurot, K. R., Broste, S. K., Frantz, R. P., . . . Hibbeln, J. R. (2016). Re-evaluation of the traditional diet-heart hypothesis: analysis of recovered data from Minnesota Coronary Experiment (1968-73). *BMJ, 353*. Retrieved from http://www.bmj.com/content/353/bmj.i1246

34 Thompson, T. (2015, February 10). U.S. Advisers Rethink Cholesterol Risk From Foods: Report. Healthday [Web log message]. Retrieved from https://consumer.healthday.com/cardiovascular-health-information-20/dietary-choloesterol-news-130/u-s-advisers-rethink-cholesterol-risk-from-foods-report-696375.html

35 Keene, D., Price, C., Shun-Shin, M. J., & Francis, D. P. (2014). Effect on cardiovascular risk of high density lipoprotein targeted drug treatments niacin, fibrates, and CETP inhibitors: meta-analysis of randomised controlled trials including 117 411 patients. *BMJ, 349*. Retrieved from http://www.bmj.com/content/349/bmj.g4379

36 Wilson, J. & Christensen, J. (2014, February 27). Nutrition labels getting a makeover. CNN [Web log message]. Retrieved from http://www.cnn.com/2014/02/27/health/nutrition-labels-changes/index.html

37 How do I get the vitamin D my body needs? (n.d.) *Vitamin D Council.* Retrieved from http://www.vitamindcouncil.org/about-vitamin-d/how-do-i-get-the-vitamin-d-my-body-needs/

38 Albrechtsson, E., Jonsson, T., Möller, S., Höglund, M., Ohlsson, B., & Axelson, J. (2003).Vitamin D receptor is expressed in pancreatic cancer cells and a vitamin D3 analogue decreases cell number. *Pancreatology, 3*(1), 41–46. Retrieved from http://www.ncbi.nlm.nih.gov/pubmed/12649563

39 Garlanda, C. F., Cuomob, R. E., Gorhama, E. D., Zenga, K., & Mohra, S. B. (2016). Cloud cover-adjusted ultraviolet B irradiance and pancreatic cancer incidence in 172 countries. *The Journal of Steroid Biochemistry and Molecular Biology, 155*(B), 257–263. Retrieved from http://www.sciencedirect.com/science/article/pii/S0960076015001016

40 Fleischer, A. & Fleischer, S. (2016). Solar radiation and the incidence and mortality of leading invasive cancers in the United States. *Dermato-Endocrinology, 8*(1), e1162366. Retrieved from http://www.ncbi.nlm.nih.gov/pmc/articles/PMC4862378/

41 Cannell, J. (2013, December 10). Why does the Vitamin D Council recommend 5,000 IU/day? [Web log message]. Vitamin D Council. Re-

trieved from https://www.vitamindcouncil.org/blog/why-does-the-vitamin-d-council-recommend-5000-iuday/

42 Yuan, C., Qian, Z. R., Babic, A., Morales-Oyarvide, V., Rubinson, D. A., Kraft, P., . . . Wolpin, B. M. (2016, June 20). Prediagnostic plasma 25-hydroxyvitamin D and pancreatic cancer survival. Journal of Clinical Oncology, Advance online publication. Retrieved from http://jco.ascopubs.org/content/early/2016/06/15/JCO.2015.66.3005.abstract

43 Gaddis, D. E., Maynard, C, L., Weaver, C. T., Michalek, S. M., & Katz, J. (2013). Role of TLR2-dependent IL-10 production in the inhibition of the initial IFN-γ T cell response to Porphyromonas gingivalis. *Journal of Leukocyte Biology, 93*(1), 21–31. Retrieved from http://www.ncbi.nlm.nih.gov/pmc/articles/PMC3525832/

44 Scutti, S. (2016, April 19). Signs of pancreatic cancer include these bacteria living in the mouth [Web log message]. Retrieved from http://www.medicaldaily.com/pancreatic-cancer-symptoms-bacteria-mouth-382505

45 Garchitorena, M. (2016, April 17). Specific mouth bacteria linked to pancreatic cancer [Web log message]. Retrieved from http://www.gastroendonews.com/Web-Only/Article/04-16/Specific-Mouth-Bacteria-Linked-to-Pancreatic-Cancer/36030/ses=ogst

46 Wang, C.-Y., Wang, H.-C., Li, J.-M., Wang, J.-Y., Yang, K.-C., Ho, Y.-K., . . . Hsueh, P.-R. (2010). Invasive infections of Aggregatibacter (Actinobacillus) actinomycetemcomitans. *Journal of Microbiology, Immunology, and Infection, 43*(6), 491–497. Retrieved from http://www.e-jmii.com/article/S1684-1182%2810%2960076-X/abstract

47 Rohrmann, S., Linseisen, J., Nöthlings, U., Overvad, K., Egeberg, R., Tjønneland, A., . . . Bueno-de-Mesquita, H. B. (2013). Meat and fish

consumption and risk of pancreatic cancer: results from the European Prospective Investigation into Cancer and Nutrition. *International Journal of Cancer, 132*(3), 617-624. Retrieved from http://onlinelibrary.wiley.com/doi/10.1002/ijc.27637/full

48 Key, T. J., Appleby, P. N., Spencer, E. A., Travis, R. C., Roddam, A. W., & Allen, N. E. (2009). Cancer incidence in vegetarians: Results from the European Prospective Investigation into Cancer and Nutrition (EPIC-Oxford). *The American Journal of Clinical Nutrition, 89*(5), 1620S-1626S. Retrieved from http://ajcn.nutrition.org/content/89/5/1620S.-long

49 Felini, M., Johnson, E., Preacely, N., Sarda, V., Ndetan, H., & Bangara, S. (2011). A pilot case-cohort study of liver and pancreatic cancers in poultry workers. *Annals of Epidemiology, 21*(10),755-66. Retrieved from http://www.ncbi.nlm.nih.gov/pubmed/21884967

50 Netto, G. F., & Johnson, E. S. (2003). Mortality in workers in poultry slaughtering/processing plants: the Missouri poultry cohort study. *Occupational and Environmental Medicine, 60*, 784-788. Retrieved from http://oem.bmj.com/content/60/10/784.full

51 Johnson, E. S. Poultry oncogenic retroviruses and humans. (1994). *Cancer Detection and Prevention, 18*(1), 9-30. Retrieved from http://www.ncbi.nlm.nih.gov/pubmed/8162609?dopt=Abstract

52 Tsang, S. X., Switzer, W. M., Shanmugam, V., Johnson, J. A., Goldsmith, C., Wright, A., . . . Heneine, W. (1999). Evidence of avian leukosis virus subgroup E and endogenous avian virus in measles and mumps vaccines derived from chicken cells: Investigation of transmission to vaccine recipients. *Journal of Virology, 73*(7), 5843-5851. Retrieved from http://jvi.asm.org/content/73/7/5843.abstractijkey=20b481e175e989349

339f668466ca114244b7707&keytype2=tf_ipsecsha

53 Pham, T. D., Spencer, J. L., Traina-Dorge, V. L., Mullin, D. A., Garry, R. F., & Johnson, E. S. (1999). Detection of exogenous and endogenous avian leukosis virus in commercial chicken eggs using reverse transcription and polymerase chain reaction assay. *Avian Pathology, 28*(4), 385-392. Retrieved from http://www.ncbi.nlm.nih.gov/pubmed/26905496

54 McGuinness, E. E., Morgan, R. G., & Wormsleyl, K. G. (1984). Effects of soybean flour on the pancreas of rats. *Environmental Health Perspectives, 56*, 205–212. Retrieved from http://www.ncbi.nlm.nih.gov/pmc/articles/PMC1568217/

55 Daniel, K. T. (n.d.). How soy wreaks havoc on digestion and the pancreas. The Healthy Home Economist [Web log message]. Retrieved from http://www.thehealthyhomeeconomist.com/not-just-bad-for-hormones-how-soy-harms-digestion-and-stresses-the-pancreas/

56 Adgent, M. A., Daniels, J. L., Rogan, W. J., Adair, L., Edwards, L. J., Westreich, D. . . . Marcus, M. (2012). Early-life soy exposure and age at menarche. *Paediatric and Perinatal Ep;idemiology, 26*(2), 163–175. Retrieved from http://onlinelibrary.wiley.com/doi/10.1111/j.1365-3016.2011.01244.x/full

57 Kim, J., Kim, S., Huh, K., Kim, Y., & Joung, H. (2011). High serum isoflavone concentrations are associated with the risk of precocious puberty in Korean girls. *Clinical Endocrinology. 75*(6), 831–835. Retrieved from http://onlinelibrary.wiley.com/doi/10.1111/j.1365-2265.2011.04127.x/full

58 Miller, Z. C. (2013, July 16). Soy products linked to cancer in lab tests: Four very convincing reasons to cut soy from your diet today [Web log message]. Natural News. Retrieved from http://www.natural-

news.com/041213_soy_warning_cancer_lab_tests.html

59 Gumbmann, M. R., Spangler, W. L., Dugan, G. M., Rackis, J. J., & Liener, I. E. (1985, September). The USDA trypsin inhibitor study. IV. The chronic effects of soy flour and soy protein isolate on the pancreas in rats after two years. *Plant Foods for Human Nutrition, 35*(3), 275–314. Retrieved from http://link.springer.com/article/10.1007/BF01092199

60 Ancira, K. (n.d.). What is the difference between sucrose, glucose & fructose? Healthy Eating [Web log message]. Retrieved from http://healthyeating.sfgate.com/difference-between-sucrose-glucose-fructose-8704.html

61 Pancreatic cancer risk factors. (2016, April, 5). American Cancer Society [Web log message] Retrieved from http://www.cancer.org/cancer/pancreaticcancer/detailedguide/pancreatic-cancer-risk-factors

62 Liu, H., Huang, D., McArthur, D. L., Boros, L. G., Nissen, N., & Heaney, A. P. (2010). Fructose induces transketolase flux to promote pancreatic cancer growth. *Cancer Research, 79*(15), 6,368–6,376. Retrieved from http://cancerres.aacrjournals.org/content/70/15/6368.long

63 Bray, G. A., Nielsen, S. J., & Popkin, B. M. (2004). Consumption of high-fructose corn syrup in beverages may play a role in the epidemic of obesity. *American Journal of Clinical Nutrition, 79*(4), 537–543. Retrieved from http://ajcn.nutrition.org/content/79/4/537.full

64 Jiao, L., Flood, A., Subar, A. F., Hollenbeck, A. R., Schatzkin, A., & Stolzenberg-Solomon, R. (2009). Glycemic index, carbohydrates, glycemic load, and the risk of pancreatic cancer in a prospective co-

hort study. *Cancer Epidemiology, Biomarkers & Prevention, 18*, 1144. Retrieved from http://cebp.aacrjournals.org/content/18/4/1144.full

65 Thiébaut, A. C. M., Jiao, L, Silverman, D. T., Cross, A. J., Thompson, F. E., Subar, A. F., . . . Rachael Z. Stolzenberg-Solomon, R. Z. (2009). Dietary fatty acids and pancreatic cancer in the NIH-AARP diet and health study. *Journal of the National Cancer Institute, 101*(14), 1001–1011. Retrieved from http://jnci.oxfordjournals.org/content/101/14/1001.full

66 Berrington de González, A., Spencer, E. A., Bueno-de-Mesquita, H. B., Roddam, A., Stolzenberg-Solomon, R., Halkjær, J., . . . Riboli, E. (2006). Anthropometry, physical activity, and the risk of pancreatic cancer in the European Prospective Investigation into Cancer and Nutrition. *Cancer Epidemiology, Biomarkers & Prevention, 15*, 879. Retrieved from http://cebp.aacrjournals.org/content/15/5/879.long

67 Aune, D., Vieira, A. R., Chan, D. S., Navarro Rosenblatt, D. A., Vieira, R., Greenwood, D. C., . . . Norat, T. (2012). Height and pancreatic cancer risk: a systematic review and meta-analysis of cohort studies. Cancer Causes and Control, 23(8), 1213-1222. Retrieved from http://www.ncbi.nlm.nih.gov/pubmed/22689322

68 Pimpin, L., Wu, J. H. Y., Haskelberg, H., Del Gobbo, L., & Mozaffarian, D. (2016). Is butter back? A systematic review and meta-analysis of butter consumption and risk of cardiovascular disease, diabetes, and total mortality. *PLoS ONE 11*(6): e0158118. Retrieved from http://journals.plos.org/plosone/article?id=10.1371%2Fjournal.pone.0158118

69 Ramsden, C. E., Zamora, D., Majchrzak-Hong, S., Faurot, K. R., Broste, S. K., Frantz, R. P., . . . Hibbeln, J. R. (2016). Re-evaluation of the traditional diet-heart hypothesis: analysis of recovered data from

Minnesota Coronary Experiment (1968-73). The BMJ 353, i1246. Retrieved from http://www.bmj.com/content/353/bmj.i1246

70 Stolzenberg-Solomon, R. Z., Schairer, C., Moore, S., Hollenbeck, A., & Silverman, D. T. (2013). Lifetime adiposity and risk of pancreatic cancer in the NIH-AARP Diet and Health Study cohort. *The American Journal of Clinical Nutrition, 98*(4), 1057-1065. Retrieved from http://ajcn.nutrition.org/content/98/4/1057.long

71 Jiao, L., Berrington de Gonzalez, A., Hartge, P., Pfeiffer, R. M., Park, Y., Freedman, D. M., . . . Stolzenberg-Solomon, R. Z. (2010). Body mass index, effect modifiers, and risk of pancreatic cancer: A pooled study of seven prospective cohorts. *Cancer Causes and Control, 21*(8), 1305–1314. Retrieved from http://www.ncbi.nlm.nih.gov/pmc/articles/PMC2904431/

72 Stolzenberg-Solomon, R. Z., Adams, K., Leitzmann, M., Schairer, C., Michaud, D. S., Hollenbeck, A., . . . Silverman, D. T. (2008). Adiposity, Physical Activity, and Pancreatic Cancer in the National Institutes of Health–AARP Diet and Health Cohort. *American Journal of Epidemiology, 167*(5), 586-597. Retrieved from http://aje.oxfordjournals.org/content/167/5/586.long

73 Jacobs, E. J., Chanock, S. J., Fuchs. C. S., LaCroix, A., McWilliams, R. R., Steplowski, E., . . . Zeleniuch-Jacquotte, A. (2010). Family history of cancer and risk of pancreatic cancer: A pooled analysis from the Pancreatic Cancer Cohort Consortium (PanScan). *International Journal of Cancer, 127*(6), 1421–1428. Retrieved from http://onlinelibrary.wiley.com/doi/10.1002/ijc.25148/full

74 Maisonneuve, P., Lowenfels, A. B., Bueno-de-Mesquita, H. B., Ghadirian, P., Baghurst, P. A., Zatonski, W. A., . . . Boyle, P. (2010). Past medical history and pancreatic cancer risk: Results from a multi-

center case-control study. *Annals of Epidemiology,20*(2), 92-98. Retrieved from http://www.ncbi.nlm.nih.gov/pubmed/20123159

75 Amundadottir, L., Kraft, P., Stolzenberg-Solomon, R. Z., Fuchs, C. S., Petersen, G. M., Arslan, A. A., . . . Hoover, R. N. (2009). Genome-wide association study identifies variants in the ABO locus associated with susceptibility to pancreatic cancer. *Nature Genetics, 41*(9), 986–990. Retrieved from http://www.ncbi.nlm.nih.gov/pmc/articles/PMC2839871/

76 Wolpin, B. M., Kraft, P., Gross, M., Helzlsouer, K., Bueno-de-Mesquita, H. B., Steplowski, E., . . . Fuchs, C. S. (2010). Pancreatic cancer risk and ABO blood group alleles: Results from the Pancreatic Cancer Cohort Consortium. *Cancer Research, 70*(3), 1015–1023. Retrieved from http://cancerres.aacrjournals.org/content/70/3/1015.long

77 Jiao, L. Silverman, D. T., Schairer, C., Thiébaut, A. C. M., Hollenbeck, A. R., Leitzmann, M., F., . . . Stolzenberg-Solomon, R. Z. (2009). Alcohol use and risk of pancreatic cancer - The NIH-AARP Diet and Health Study. *American Journal of Epidemiology, 169*(9), 1043-1051. Retrieved from http://aje.oxfordjournals.org/content/169/9/1043.long

78 Bao, Y., Stolzenberg-Solomon, R., Jiao, L., Silverman, D. T., Subar, A. F., Park, Y., . . . Michaud, D. S. (2008). Added sugar and sugar-sweetened foods and beverages and the risk of pancreatic cancer in the National Institutes of Health–AARP Diet and Health Study. *The American Journal of Clinical Nutrition, 88*(2), 431-440. Retrieved from http://ajcn.nutrition.org/content/88/2/431.long

79 Guertin, K. A., Freedman, N. D., Loftfield, E., Stolzenberg-Solomon, R. Z., Graubard, B., & Sinha, R, (2015). A prospective study of coffee intake and pancreatic cancer: results from the NIH-AARP Diet and Health Study. *British Journal of Cancer, 113*(7), 1081-1085. Retrieved from http://www.ncbi.nlm.nih.gov/pubmed/26402414

80 Gardner, T. B. (n.d.). Pancreatic neuroendocrine tumors [Web log message]. The National Pancreas Foundation. Retrieved from https://www.pancreasfoundation.org/patient-information/pancreatic-cancer/pancreatic-neuroendocrine-tumors/

81 McDougall, J. (2011, November). Why did Steve Jobs die? The McDougall Newsletter [Web log message]. Retrieved from https://www.drmcdougall.com/misc/2011nl/nov/jobs.htm

82 Mertz, R. (2014, January 6). Did you know that Steve Jobs became vegan because he believed the diet would... [Web log message]. Retrieved from http://www.tydknow.com/did-you-know-that-steve-jobs-became-vegan-because-he-believed-the-diet-would/

83 Daniel, K. (2011, December 27). iVegetarian2: The eating disorders of Steve Jobs. The Weston A. Price Foundation [Web log message]. Retrieved from http://www.westonaprice.org/health-topics/soy-alert/ivegetarian2-the-eating-disorders-of-steve-jobs/

84 Dahl, M. (2011, November 2). The strange eating habits of Steve Jobs. NBC News [Web log message]. Retrieved from http://www.nbc-news.com/health/body-odd/strange-eating-habits-steve-jobs-f119434

85 Bruso, J. (2015, May 1). What are the effects of a fat deficiency in humans? Livestrong.com [Web log message]. Retrieved from http://www.livestrong.com/article/503785-what-are-the-effects-of-fat-deficiencies-in-humans/

86 Axe, J. (2011). Steve Jobs: His treatment plan, where it went wrong [Web log message]. Retrieved from https://draxe.com/steve-jobs-twenty-year-battle-with-pancreatic-cancer/

87 Verma, R.,Foster, R. E., Horgan, K., Mounsey, K., Nixon, H., Smalle, N., . . . Carter, C. R. D. (2016, January 26). Lymphocyte depletion and

repopulation after chemotherapy for primary breast cancer. BioMed Central, 18(10). Advance online publication. Retrieved from http://breast-cancer-research.biomedcentral.com/articles/10.1186/s13058-015-0669-x

88 Altman, L. K., & Wade, N. (2011, October 3). One of 3 chosen for Nobel in medicine died days ago. The New York Times [Web log message]. Retrieved from http://www.nytimes.com/2011/10/04/science/04nobel.html?_r=0

89 Gravitz, L. (2011, October 11). A fight for life that united a field. Nature, 478, 163–164. Retrieved from http://www.nature.com/news/2011/111012/full/478163a.html

90 Engber, D. (2012, December 21). Is the cure for cancere inside you? The New York Times Magazine [Web log message]. Retrieved from http://www.nytimes.com/2012/12/23/magazine/is-the-cure-for-cancer-inside-you.html

91 Cancer Research Institute. (n.d.). Ralph Steinman on Dendritic Cells and Cancer Immunotherapy [Web log message]. Retrieved from http://www.cancerresearch.org/our-strategy-impact/people-be-hind-the-progress/scientists/ralph-steinman

92 Revising the Timeline for Deadly Pancreatic Cancer. (2010, October 27). HHMI News. Howard Hughes Medical Institute. Retrieved from http://www.hhmi.org/news/revising-timeline-deadly-pancreatic-cancer

93 Yachida, S., Jones, S., Bozic, I., Antal, T., Leary, R., Fu, B., . . . Iacobuzio-Donahue C. A. (2010).Distant metastasis occurs late during the genetic evolution of pancreatic cancer. *Nature, 467*, 1114–1117. Retrieved from http://www.nature.com/nature/journal/v467/n7319/full/nature09515.h

tml

94 Ranjan, A. P., Mukerjee, A., Helson, L., Gupta, R., & Vishwanatha, J. K. (2013). Efficacy of liposomal curcumin in a human pancreatic tumor xenograft model: inhibition of tumor growth and angiogenesis. *Anticancer Research, 33*(9), 3603-2609. Retrieved from http://ar.iiarjournals.org/content/33/9/3603.long

95 Dhillon, N., Aggarwal, B. B., Newman, R. A., Wolff, R. A., Kunnumakkara, A. B., Abbruzzese, J. L., . . . Razelle Kurzrock, R. (2008).Phase II Trial of Curcumin in patients with advanced pancreatic cancer. *Clinical Cancer Research, 14*(14), 4491–4499. Retrieved from http://clincancerres.aacrjournals.org/content/14/14/4491

96 Kanai, M. (2014). Therapeutic applications of curcumin for patients with pancreatic cancer. *World Journal of Gastroenterology, 20*(28), 9384–9391. Retrieved from http://www.ncbi.nlm.nih.gov/pmc/articles/PMC4110570/

97 Mulcahy, N. (2016, June 4). In pancreatic cancer, a 'step' means a new standard of care. Medscape [Web log message]. Retrieved from http://www.medscape.com/viewarticle/864313?src=WNL_confalert_160604_MSCPEDIT

98 Satija, A., Bhupathiraju, S. N., Rimm, E. B., Spiegelman, D., Chiuve, S. E., Borgi, L, . . . Hu, F. B. (2016). Plant-based dietary patterns and incidence of Type 2 diabetes in US men and women: Results from three prospective cohort studies. *PLoS Med 13*(6), e1002039. Retrieved from http://journals.plos.org/plosmedicine/article?id=10.1371/journal.pmed.1002039

99 Rumawas, M. E., McKeown, N. M., Rogers, G., Meigs, J. B., Wilson, P. W., & Jacques, P. F. (2006). Magnesium intake is related to improved insulin homeostasis in the framingham offspring cohort. *The Journal*

of the American College of Nutrition, 25(6), 486-492. Retrieved from http://www.ncbi.nlm.nih.gov/pubmed/17229895

100Lin, B-H, & Morrison, R. M. (2016, July 5). A closer look at declining fruit and vegetable consumption using linked data sources. Amber Waves. USDA Economic Research Service [Web log message]. Retrieved from http://www.ers.usda.gov/amber-waves/2016-july/a-closer-look-at-declining-fruit-and-vegetable-consumption-using-linked-data-sources.aspx#.V6O9OaJEjgb

101Wang, J. (2015, February 2). Colon cancer linked to viruses in beef, Nobel-winning scientist contends. Health. South China Morning Post [Web log message]. Retrieved from http://www.scmp.com/lifestyle/health/article/1695757/colon-cancer-linked-viruses-beef-nobel-winning-scientist-contends

102Bulajic, M., Panic, N., & Löhr, J. M. (2014). Helicobacter pylori and pancreatic diseases. *World Journal of Gastrointestinal Pathophysiology, 5*(4), 380–383. http://www.ncbi.nlm.nih.gov/pmc/articles/PMC4231501/

Printed in Great Britain
by Amazon

12976479R00071